Glen R. Elliott, Ph.D., M.D.
Director, The Children's Center at Langley Porter
University of California, San Francisco

with KATE KELLY

MEDICATING YOUNG MINDS

How to Know If Psychiatric Drugs
Will Help or Hurt Your Child

A Lynn Sonberg Book

STC HEALTHY LIVING
Stewart, Tabori & Chang
NEW YORK

Editor: Christine Gardner
Designer: woolypear
Production Manager: Jane Searle

Library of Congress Cataloging-in-Publication Data
Glen R. Elliott; with Kate Kelly.
  Medicating young minds : how to know if psychiatric drugs will help or hurt your child / Glen R. Elliott.
      p. cm.
  Includes index.
  ISBN 1-58479-489-5
  1. Pediatric psychopharmacology--Popular works. 2. Behavior disorders in children--Chemotherapy--Popular works.
  3. Child psychopathology--Chemotherapy--Popular works. I. Title.

RJ504.7.E55 2006
618.92'8918--dc22   2006001866

Published in 2006 by Stewart, Tabori & Chang
An imprint of Harry N. Abrams, Inc.

The text of this book was composed in Ocra, Kepler, and Trade Gothic Condensed.

Printed and bound in the United States of America.
10 9 8 7 6 5 4 3 2 1

HNA ■■■■■
harry n. abrams, inc.
a subsidiary of La Martinière Groupe
115 West 18th Street
New York, NY 10011
www.hnabooks.com

Disclaimer
This book is intended as a reference guide, not as a medical guide or manual for self-treatment. The information is
intended to help you make informed decisions. The recommendations in this book should be used only with the consent
of your doctor. Do not make any changes in treatment without consulting with and getting the consent of your doctor.

To the patients and families
who are the motivation for and basis of this work

and

to my wife and children, Jan, James, and Mark,
who keep me grounded

. . . .

Contents

Introduction

The majority of us think of childhood and adolescence as a happy, almost carefree time. However, a combination of research and public education over the past twenty years has helped to disabuse us of this fantasy. We now know that between 12 and 22 percent of children in the United States have marked problems that fall under the category of mental or psychiatric illness. This includes a wide range of difficulties, from severe delays in normal development such as mental retardation and autism, to emotional and behavioral disturbances including depression, attention-deficit/hyperactivity disorder (ADHD), and anxiety.

Sadly, most children and adolescents with severe psychiatric disorders and behavioral problems still remain undiagnosed, and an estimated 80 percent of them receive no mental health care of any kind. Clearly, we need to do more to provide effective diagnosis and treatment. One promising approach to helping some of these young people is the use of what are often called psychoactive medications; that is, medicines that alter how the brain works in ways that change mood, behavior, and thinking.

Parents facing the possibility of giving such medications to their child, however, are often understandably and justifiably hesitant to do so. Physicians who prescribe these types of medicines often tend to downplay risks and emphasize potential benefits. Yet many other sources of information would have you believe that using a psychoactive medication is the moral equivalent of giving your child rat poison. Even the U.S. government got into the act. In 2004, the Food and Drug Administration (FDA) demanded that manufacturers of ten popular antidepressants add or strengthen the suicide-related warnings on their labels, specifically focusing on use by children and adolescents. And in early 2005, newspapers trumpeted Canada's decision to ban a popular stimulant, Adderall XR (used to treat ADHD), because of evidence suggesting it has the potential to cause sudden death. Canada's reversal of that decision later that same year, after reviewing the evidence, went largely unheralded.

As both a parent and a professional, I am well aware that no one chooses to have a child who suffers from a psychiatric disorder. Similarly, I know we all want to have health insurance for ourselves and our families. And yet, most of us never even think to inquire about mental health coverage for our children—until we need it. Then, of course, it's often too late.

Similarly, you are reading this book because, suddenly and largely unexpectedly, you realize that your child may have a serious psychiatric disorder or behavioral problem. Someone has told you that your child's problems are so severe that you should think about "putting him on medicine." And, just that quickly, you find yourself trying to sort through a welter of uncertainties, conflicting information, and false promises of cures. I know, because I see these families in my office every day.

In the middle of all this family chaos is a child whose brain and body are still developing, whose social skills are being formed, whose emotional framework is being assembled, and whose educational needs must be met. When psychiatric medications are introduced into the picture—drugs whose very purpose is to alter the way the brain functions—it's understandable that parents are reluctant to face this prospect. It's also understandable why many parents who have a child who is completely disrupting family life and the school environment are more than eager to give the child something that will at least alleviate some of the disruptive behavior.

It is my desire to give parents of troubled children a broader vision of psychiatric illness as it affects young individuals, as well as a view of what we know—and what we don't—about the psychoactive drugs that may play a role in treatment. Such medications can literally save a child's life, but they can also worsen problems or create entirely new ones.

When I was a child, my mother loved teaching me clichés and the lessons that lay within them, particularly those with contradictory meanings. I find myself thinking of some that are relevant to this discussion: "Desperate times call for desperate measures," but "haste makes waste." And "nothing ventured, nothing gained" may or may not trump "fools rush in where angels fear to tread." What I want to convey to all parents is the message that the decisions you are being asked to make are, indeed, as serious as they feel to you.

You may well find this book disquieting. Seldom will I offer an unequivocal statement, except for this: Beware of the "quick fix." I know all too well how difficult it can be to take it slow, especially in a crisis. However, I have found that once a family realizes someone is taking them seriously, they start to relax—even before I do anything else. By buying this bit of extra time for everyone, I hope to gain the opportunity to more fully evaluate the situation so that the best remedy can be found.

It is my hope that this book will also calm and reassure you as you make the difficult decision whether or not to give psychiatric medications to your child, and how to continue to nurture and help your child, whatever your choices may be.

A Bit About Myself

I entered medical school in the early 1970s wanting to study psychiatry and understand the chemistry of the brain. By the time I had obtained both a Ph.D. and an M.D., I was still committed to psychiatry but had gained a much better appreciation of the complexity of the brain and how little we understand about its function. At the same time, my fascination with the ways in which relatively simple compounds can alter brain systems continued to grow.

I came to child and adolescent psychiatry relatively late in my training and somewhat by happenstance. Child and adolescent psychiatrists must first finish medical school (usually a matter of four or five years after college, but in my case seven years because of the concurrent Ph.D.). Then they must complete three or four years of residency training in general psychiatry, which focuses largely on adults. After that, there is an additional two years of specialty training, working specifically with younger patients and their families.

I managed to spread the whole training process out over fourteen years by doing mental health policy work in Washington, D.C., for a year in the midst of my other training. My parents began to wonder if I'd ever be anything but a student!

When I entered child and adolescent psychiatry training in the mid-1980s, I brought along my interest in psychopharmacology, the study of drugs that affect the brain and behavior. It was both a wonderfully exciting and incredibly frustrating time to combine the two fields. There were well under a hundred papers and exactly two textbooks written about child and adolescent psychopharmacology, so it didn't take long to master the available knowledge—or to appreciate just how little we knew. The literature is considerably more voluminous and sophisticated now, and yet it only seems to emphasize how much we have yet to learn.

Since 1989, I have been director of the Children's Center at Langley Porter, which is the home for child and adolescent psychiatry at the University of California, San Francisco. We train child and adolescent psychiatrists, general psychiatry residents, and medical students. We conduct research to try to find better ways of identifying childhood mental disorders, as well as preventing and treating them. We also provide patient care.

My practice encompasses a huge variety of cases from mild to severe, but my particular interest is in young patients with complex, difficult-to-treat mood or behavior disorders on whom others have given up. What is the root of these disorders? Why has medicine failed to work? What else can we try? In this book, you will meet quite a few of the young people I have treated—the so-called "easy" cases, as well as the more difficult ones—although I have changed their names and disguised their backgrounds to maintain their privacy. I want to share the invaluable lessons that they and their families have taught me over the years.

. . . .
How to Use This Book
. . . .

While I know there will be a strong temptation to turn quickly to the section of the book that you believe pertains to your child, I urge you to read through Part Two first. In this section I demystify the medical process and offer suggestions for how you can find a medical professional you can trust. I also describe in detail the process you and your child will experience when undergoing a thorough evaluation. These chapters also explain some of the controversies surrounding psychiatric medications, making you better informed about the benefits as well as the possible drawbacks that can arise.

Part Two provides an explanation of the disorders themselves. After reading this section, you will have a better understanding of your child's behavior. I also offer guidelines (further explored in the next two parts of the book) about what you can do about it.

Part Three begins with an important introduction that is required reading for any family whose child is going on medication. While the drugs themselves are explained in the appropriate chapters, this section discusses a range of general issues that confront all parents considering psychoactive medications for a child, including how to talk with your child about his or her need for medications, gaining his or her cooperation, and working with their school regarding dispensing the medication.

In Part Four, you will find additional helpful information—from nondrug therapies to what you need to know about working with your child's school. These chapters will offer help to all, regardless of your child's diagnosis.

There is a lot of information to absorb, so I hope you'll read through Part One first and then whatever sections that seem most relevant to your child's problems. Then keep the book nearby as you go through the evaluation process—as additional questions arise, you'll find it helpful to refer to the book again and again.

Most of all, I want to assure you that

you need not face the problems your child is having alone. Help is available, and change is possible. But you need to be an informed consumer so you can partner with a professional who has the tools to help your son or daughter and your whole family. This book will provide you with the tools you'll need if psychoactive medications are likely to be part of the solution.

Dr. Glen R. Elliott
Director, The Children's Center at Langley Porter, University of California, San Francisco
March 2006

PART ONE

Beginning to Take Control

. . . .

Chapter 1

Children and Psychiatric Drugs: What We Know, What We Don't, and Why

. . . .

If you're considering the possibility that your child may need medication for a mood or behavior disorder, you are not alone. More and more children in the United States are being prescribed psychiatric medications—for attention-deficit/ hyperactivity disorder (ADHD), anxiety disorders, depression, bipolar disorder, and psychotic disorders, along with a host of "bad behaviors," such as aggression, tantrums, and excessive moodiness, to name a few. Prescriptions for children and adolescents with such problems doubled, and in some cases tripled, during a ten-year period (1987 through 1996), according to a study published in the *Archives of Pediatrics and Adolescent Medicine.*

In my office, I repeatedly face a variety of family attitudes about medications in general, and medications for children in particular. One family wants a "magic pill" that will make all their child's problems disappear, and they totally dismiss the possibility that medicines can have unwanted side effects. Another family knows their child needs medicine but is so overly focused on side effects that they cannot agree to proceed. Yet another family brings in a child who is on four or five different medicines at the same time— and ask me to add another because he's "not doing well."

Recently, a family came to my office. Their son, Tim, has a long history of severe behavioral problems both at home and at school. The parents explained to me that they had resisted seeking psychiatric advice for several years, despite major disruptions in their family life. Tim's fourth-grade teacher, however, had just called them in for their third conference in less than two months and told them that unless he "got help," he would not pass and would probably be expelled from school.

"You won't have to put Tim on medication, will you?" asked his mother. My answer, without yet knowing the source of his problem, was, "First, he must be carefully evaluated, and only then if we all agree that's the best answer."

In sharp contrast to Tim's situation was another family who recently visited my office. "Hyperactive" does not quite do justice to their six-year-old, who proceeded to try to open every drawer and explore every cranny in my office as his parents described why they had come. On the second day of school, he had thrown a tantrum in his first-grade class and been sent to the principal. The principal had left the boy in his office while stepping outside to speak with the teacher. He returned to find the boy stark naked, urinating on his desk and computer. Almost the first words out of his mother's mouth were, "What can you give him, Dr. Elliott? We need something that will help right away."

It is essential for everyone—family members and medical professional—to come to a mutual agreement about what the problem is and why it might be occurring. Not infrequently, some family members want to try a medication in an effort to give a child relief from a difficult problem, while other family members are still resistant. This can be especially difficult in families where there has been a divorce. Only after everyone agrees can we move toward finding the most helpful intervention, and determine whether or not medication should be considered.

The next step is working out a plan. Should the family try a form of therapy other than medicine first, or is medication an appropriate early step? If so, exactly which medicine, and how will your child be monitored as to dosage, efficacy, and possible side effects? As you'll learn, there is a systematic manner to this process that greatly increases the likelihood of a good outcome.

No Easy Answers

Widespread recognition of psychiatric disorders in children and adolescents is a relatively new phenomenon. The subspecialty of child and adolescent psychiatry is only a bit more than fifty years old, and doctors have spent much of that time convincing themselves, and others, that children are not just a product of their environment. As important as good parenting and a protective, supportive, and stimulating upbringing are, it isn't enough to guarantee a happy, well-functioning, mentally healthy child. As a society, and certainly as parents, we have become aware—some would even argue too aware—that our children are vulnerable.

But with that awareness comes a new issue: What, exactly, is the problem, and what can we do about it? At least when parents—let's be honest, mothers—were thought to be the ultimate source of most of a child's problems, the answer seemed straightforward, if simplistic: Give the child a better mother, directly or indirectly. Now, parents feel guilty for other reasons. Your child doesn't mix well with peers, has tantrums, or is "strong-willed." Does he have a disorder? If so, what is it? What do you do about it? What happens if you wait too long?

Now another problem arises: We have everyone's attention, but no one can agree on what to do next. Diagnosing psychiatric disorders in children and adolescents is often far from easy. We have no specific blood tests, brain scans, or any other procedure guaranteed to give us an unequivocal answer to any given child's "real" problem. Instead, we must rely on what we see and hear during clinical visits and learn from taking a history to try to fit each child into the right diagnostic box, and the definition of who belongs in each box can change over time.

Efforts to convey information to parents sometimes just adds to the confusion. In my professional lifetime, I have seen a series of books about a core cluster of problematic young children who are difficult to parent, easily overwhelmed, impossible with peers, rageful, and vindictive. Depending on the book and the spirit of the times, these children are labeled "strong-willed," "ADHD," "borderline," or "bipolar."

Adding to this confusion is a tangle of largely unproven therapies, each of which makes extravagant claims about who needs them and how well they work. Play therapy, floor time, cognitive therapy, behavior therapy, holding therapy, auditory therapy, nutritional therapy, homeopathy—the list seems endless, and each has it proponents and the inevitable poster child of success.

I am, unabashedly, a child and adolescent psychopharmacologist. As I explained in the Introduction, I became a physician focused on psychiatry because of a fascination with brain chemistry. When I entered child and adolescent psychiatry in the mid-1980s, the use of medications to treat severe childhood mental disorders was, pardon the pun, in its infancy. There was an infectious optimism that psychoactive medications offered not only *an* answer for many of the problems plaguing children, but *the* answer. And indeed—medications can be helpful, sometimes enormously so. However, the expectation that medicine can alleviate any and all difficulties is impossibly naive, especially when we can't always agree on what it is we're treating.

All too often, my patients start as labels rather than children. Parents come in asking for treatment for "ADHD"

NO SHORTCUTS

Pauline and Jack came to me looking for a "magic bullet" for their eleven-year-old daughter, Karleen, who had been "the perfect child" at home and at school until a few months before her eleventh birthday. That's when her grades started to slide and her teacher sent home a note stating that Karleen wasn't paying attention in class and had stopped participating. At home, their once talkative, cheerful child was moody and unresponsive, giving monosyllabic answers to questions and locking herself in her room for hours.

Pauline and Jack were confused and upset with their daughter's behavior and took her to the pediatrician, asking if he could "do something." He said Karleen was depressed and prescribed fluoxetine (Prozac), a popular antidepressant generally prescribed for adults. Within days Karleen began to have trouble sleeping, and had no improvement in her mood. Over the next few weeks, her inability to get to sleep and stay asleep grew worse. When Pauline complained about this problem to the pediatrician over the phone, he prescribed clonidine, a highly sedating drug used mainly to decrease high blood pressure, which some physicians also use to counteract medication-induced sleep problems. When Karleen had a panic attack, Pauline and Jack panicked too. That's when the pediatrician suggested keeping Karleen on clonidine but taking her off fluoxetine and switching to another antidepressant. Again, he did all this over the phone. It's also when Pauline and Jack wisely decided to seek a second opinion and came to my office.

Although many parents search for easy, quick answers, their quests are often in vain. There are no miracle cures or quick fixes for children who have mood or behavioral problems, nor are there any shortcuts. I wish I could assure you that none of my patients have had the poor response to medications that Karleen did—I can't. Bad things happen even under the best of circumstances. However, knowing that you are embarking on a complicated journey is a key first step. The parents who are active participants in the diagnosis and treatment of their child are likely to see the most positive results.

or "obsessive-compulsive disorder (OCD)" or "depression" or, especially lately, "bipolar disorder." When I ask about the basis of their diagnosis, I generally hear that the teacher or the pediatrician told them, or that the parent read a book or saw an article on the Internet that describes the child perfectly. Sometimes parents think they can just come in to pick up a prescription that "will make things better." Such parents are inevitably surprised (and not infrequently resistant initially) when they learn that I want to know a great deal more about them and their child, rather than what everyone else thinks is wrong.

Changing Attitudes Toward Mental Health Issues

In 2003, I was quoted in *Time* magazine on the subject of psychiatric medications. "The problem is that our usage has outstripped our knowledge base. Let's face it: We're experimenting on these kids without tracking the results," were among my comments at the time.

Since then, a lot has changed in the field of metal health, but, as you'll see, we're still operating without definitive guidelines for the majority of medications we routinely prescribe for children and adolescents. Let me be clear: I am not calling for more mandatory guidelines. The problem is lack of knowledge, not lack of regulations.

The good news first: There is a new awareness of the importance of issues surrounding mental well-being. We are seeing changes on both the federal and the state levels and, partly as a result of these changes, health insurance companies are being held accountable for covering mental illness in new ways (although there is still a major need for improvement). On the federal level, new mental health guidelines have just recently been passed, meaning that mental health evaluations will become more routine. In addition, the appropriations bill that passed at the end of 2004 set aside $20 million for states to overhaul their mental health programs, further expanding the reach of these new guidelines.

Many states have also passed so-called "parity" laws, insisting that insurance companies must provide coverage for major mental disorders at a level comparable to that which other illnesses receive. (Unfortunately, this often leads to the practice of "carve-out," in which the insurance company contracts another provider for mental health services—with coverage still far from adequate. Due to this practice, children and adolescents seem especially likely to receive minimal to no effective coverage.) In California, voters passed a special tax in 2005 providing hundreds of millions of dollars each year to care for underserved populations and to train more mental health care professionals. Hopefully, some fraction of that will go toward serving mentally ill children.

Our nation is also undergoing a major change in attitude towards psychoactive medications—drugs that target the brain with the intent of changing behavior and cognitive processes. Instead of viewing patients who take these medications as "crazy" or "weak," the general public increasingly sees these medications as reasonable solutions for people who have mood or behavior disorders. Even before the federal mandate to screen more children for mental health issues was instituted, there was a noticeable increase in the number of children on such medications. The number of children on psychoactive medicines jumped 20 percent from 2000 to 2003, according to Medco Health Solutions, Inc. Data—and spending on medications for treating ADHD increased threefold for children under five during that period. At the same time, and certainly not coincidentally, the number of patients thought to be responsive to psychoactive medications—those with ADHD, anxiety, depression, and bipolar disorder—skyrocketed.

Then came news that linked antidepressant medications and a possible increase in teenage suicides. Regardless of what the research said, the press was intent on broadcasting this story: By giving your child medication, you might cause him to kill himself. Even more recently, there have been stories of sudden death from Adderall—a type of stimulant used to treat ADHD—causing Canada to briefly ban its use. Another study that caused alarm concerns Ritalin (also used to treat ADHD). The authors suggested its use could cause DNA breakdown, resulting in an increased risk of cancer. Suddenly, parents and other physicians were calling me, asking for advice. Were we harming our children by trying to help them?

. . . .
The Truth Behind the Headlines
. . . .

Headlines are designed to grab our attention; they do not always represent great truths or great science. So what is a parent to think when they read news stories indicating that these medications are "bad news"? Typically, these reports are based on limited data, sometimes just a single case. After a pair of youths killed twelve students and a teacher at Columbine High School in Littleton, Colorado, reporters discovered that at least one of the perpetrators had been on an antidepressant. I got a flood of calls from journalists asking if that could be why he committed such a horrible act. Most reporters were frustrated with my reply, which was, "Maybe, but probably not," and they especially did not like my asking them how his taking a medication could explain why his friend had committed the same acts. I did not get my name in print that week.

Doctors cannot offer prescriptive advice or meaningful comments about diagnosis or motivation when all they know about an individual is what they have read in the newspaper. I did not have detailed information about that youth, and available research on the medication he was taking tells us little about the likelihood of such an event. It is quite possible that someone gave the teenager an antidepressant with the hope of *averting* such an outcome. The fact that it didn't work could be the result of many factors, from having chosen the wrong type of medication or the wrong dosage, to the medicine simply not working. Perhaps no medication would have worked—maybe his motivations to commit that horrendous act had nothing to do with a psychiatric disorder. There is a possibility that the medication caused an undetected manic episode that resulted in violence, but none of the limited information available seemed to suggest that had occurred. But while indefinable responses do not make headlines, this kind of nuanced attention to the possibilities does make good medical practice.

On the other hand, headlines can precipitate action. A suicide by a college student during a clinical trial of duloxetine (Cymbalta), one of the newest antidepressants available in the U.S., occurred at the same time the FDA was reviewing large volumes of data about antidepressants. The FDA had already begun to inquire about the effects of antidepressants on young patients based on news from Britain, where the use of all antidepressants except fluoxetine (Prozac) for children and adolescents was banned in 2004. (In 1993 and again in 2000, Britain issued warnings about the potential dangers of another type of antidepressant, selective serotonin reuptake inhibitors [SSRIs].)

In early 2004, the FDA convened a panel to discuss suicide as a possible side effect of antidepressants in children and adolescents. (Interestingly, although the evidence strongly suggests that children and adults have similar reactions to antidepressants, the question was limited to young patients.) The panel concluded that the possibility for suicide in these patients exists, but recommended a more careful analysis of available data. As a result, the FDA granted access to all available antidepressant drug trials in children and adolescents to a group from Columbia University that reviewed all reports of suicidal thoughts or attempts. The group found that no completed suicides occurred among children or adolescents in any of these studies, and they failed to find any evidence of differences among suicidal tendencies among the antidepressants they studied. There was only a slight suggestion of an increased risk of such ideas or behaviors during the first ten days of starting medication.

The FDA considered these findings and the information currently available and decided to require pharmaceutical companies to strengthen their standard cautions to patients by placing a "black box" warning label on all antidepressants starting in February 2005. These warning labels assert that the drugs increase the risk of suicidal thoughts and behaviors in children and adolescents taking them, particularly early in treatment. The effect of the above events on physicians and the general public was marked. Over the course of 2004, the number of patients under the age of eighteen taking these drugs dropped notably—this was even more remarkable given the steady increases during previous years. Medco Health Solutions, Inc. reports a full 10 percent drop in usage, after an increase of almost the same amount in 2003.

In early 2006, the FDA also began considering a "black-box warning" for stimulants (both methylphenidate and amphetamine) because of concerns that individuals taking these drugs might be at risk of sudden death from disruptions of heart function. Previous assessments of this risk had not led to a specific warning, as the likelihood of death was thought to be one or two per million. It remains unclear whether the FDA believes that such a rare but deadly risk actually exists for this class or medications and, if so, what course of action is needed. What was clear was that the decision process was as much political as scientific.

So What Does All This Mean for Your Child?

Whether the changes I just described are good or bad for you and your child depends on your point of view. I find the whole chain of events upsetting. Throughout the 1990s and early 2000s, I expended considerable effort pleading with colleagues not to assume that "relatively safe" meant "risk free." Children should not be receiving medications they don't need. But I am equally upset by the overreaction to data when it finally became available. Are we to conclude that the 10 percent of children no longer taking antidepressants should never have been on them? Or, given the very real risks of untreated depression or incapacitating anxiety, are they now being penalized because of a low (but possibly real) risk of hurting themselves? I can only hope that, at the very least, the patients were weaned off their antidepressants gradually, because abruptly stopping the taking of medicines can be as risky as starting them in the first place.

As a result of all this new information, physicians are now expected to tell patients and families something about side effects if they recommend an antidepressant. But what, exactly? That the very medicine they are suggesting carries a small risk of making your child worse? How much worse? How big a risk? It's a bit like a forecaster predicting a 3 percent chance of rain. Should I stay home to avoid getting wet? Am I less wet if I go out and get caught in a downpour? How do I make a reasoned decision, especially if I am—or worse—my child is in a crisis?

Another problem these findings create relates to who provides care. Many pediatricians and general practitioners, the primary prescribers for most antidepressants in young patients, have grown wary of the potential risks of using this important class of drugs. As a result, kids who need treatment may be told "let's wait and see," when they might feel better if they received appropriate medications. And, as we will discuss in Chapter 5, untreated depression carries an all-too-real risk of suicidal ideation, attempts, and completion.

We're in a quandary. Both doing nothing and doing something can be devastating. Both the failure to use medications and their inappropriate use can have a significant impact on children's lives and be detrimental to their health, welfare, and future. However, there is a solution. What we need is preliminary mental health screening done by pediatricians or schools. Then, children and adolescents who show signs of mental health problems should be carefully evaluated and treatment options explored. If medications seem in order, young patients should be monitored carefully by the prescribing professional to reduce the risk of giving them the wrong drug.

How Medicines for Children Are Tested and Approved

Here is a little-known but crucial fact: It is a common practice for doctors to prescribe medication for treating ailments other than those approved for the drug—often with little or no information about its long-term safety. This is especially true for children and adolescents. Check the inserts pharmacists are supposed to give you when you get a new prescription—have you ever actually read one? You will almost invariably find a phrase such as, "This medication has not been proven to be safe and effective in individuals under age sixteen" (or eighteen, or even in children or adolescents).

FDA approval of a medication requires that a pharmaceutical company establish the safety and efficacy of the drug at a specific range of doses in a specific age group for a specific disorder. For the most part, companies choose to study adults, not younger patients. This is true across all of fields of medicine, but especially for psychiatry.

In addition to alternate uses, it is also important to be aware that not all medications have been approved according to the same standards. Currently, all medications must pass a review for safety and efficacy for a specific condition before the FDA will endorse their sale in the U.S. Medications in use before the 1970s, when FDA developed these more rigorous standards, were "grandfathered in" and assumed to be safe and effective. Thus many older medications, some of which have a wide array of serious side effects, are being given to children as young as two, not because of testing, but because they were already in widespread use. This leads physicians and families to another quandary: Should they use older medications with known, sometimes worrisome side effects or new medications that, while not specifically tested in children, appear to be effective and safe in adults, based on fairly short-term studies?

At least for now, physicians are allowed to use any FDA-endorsed drug in whatever way they deem beneficial, as long as there is some evidence that it could be helpful. Such use is called "off-label." Although physicians are strongly encouraged to inform families when a drug is being prescribed off-label, the reality is that nearly all recent psychoactive medications used in young patients are off-label.

Why do doctors prescribe medication approved for one disorder or illness for a different illness? Because small experiments and anecdotal evidence says it works. For example, experience has taught us that many anticonvulsants (drugs that help control epileptic seizures) are also effective in treating bipolar disorder. As a result, when a new anticonvulsant becomes available, some clinicians will begin testing it as a mood stabilizer, mostly in adults. If the medication seems to help, the clinician may publish what is called a case report, or

may simply tell colleagues, who pass it on to other colleagues. Word spreads, and others begin using it. Inevitably, it starts being used in children and adolescents too. Since some mood stabilizers also help with violent behaviors and other common conditions that have nothing to do with bipolar disorder, a new drug thought to be a good mood stabilizer may quickly become widely used for many other conditions—all without any true research. This type of work, often just clinical reports based on a few patients, is much simpler, faster, and far cheaper than what the FDA requires. However, it also is plagued with uncertainties about genuine efficacy and safety.

Another problem is that there is no single repository of information about calibrating drug dosages for children. Turn to the *Physicians' Desk Reference* (PDR), an omnipresent tool in doctors' offices that offers a complete set of guidelines and warnings supplied by drug companies, for example. There is little, if any, information on how certain drugs affect children. Unfortunately, bad experiences have proven that children are not just little adults. There have been tragic examples of adult dosages of certain medications being adjusted to allow for a child's smaller size, with no consideration for the different ways in which children's organs may process the medication. This has resulted in seizures, shock, and even death.

The reason for this information gap is twofold: First, full-scale studies and clinical trials are costly. In recent years, federal legislation has sought to give financial incentives to pharmaceutical firms to sponsor clinical studies targeting children. One such incentive gives drug companies a six-month extension of market exclusivity for a medication if they agree to set up a pediatric trial to screen it. Still, that scarcely begins to address the cost.

Fear has been another reason companies don't test drugs on children. In the 1950s and '60s—before we became such a litigious society—cancer medications were actually tested on children before being used on adults. Today, companies would never use children as guinea pigs, nor are they totally comfortable with running the types of clinical trials they would on adults. There is concern both about the degree to which children should have a say in whether or not they participate and whether parental consent is enough protection for the child. Drug companies are very nervous about the possibility of being sued if something goes wrong. Jury awards can be quite high under these circumstances.

Realistically, I cannot offer a universal answer to the dilemma families face when a doctor recommends a psychoactive medication for their child. In my experience, the only time medications seem blemish-free is when they are first released; only then do they seem perfectly safe and effective. In truth, I typically discourage the use of new medications, especially in children, for at least several months, so that more experience with adults can help to inform us about possible advantages and risks.

Families need to understand that de-

THE PEDIATRIC RULE

In 2003, the U.S. Congress passed the Pediatric Rule, which specifies that pediatric studies must be included when investigating any medications that might be used for conditions that affect both adults and children. While this reform is a step in the right direction, we still have no process for testing medications that are already on the market or for evaluating whether or not a generic medication acts on a child exactly as the brand-name version it is replacing. The FDA's method for monitoring drugs already available is a passive one, where doctors voluntarily fill out paperwork reporting adverse effects suffered by any patient on a certain medication. Any parent who has spent time in a hectic pediatrician's office will realize that the odds are not good that a doctor will have time to do this extra paperwork.

ciding to start medicating is a joint decision between the doctor and the family. The physician promises to provide the best available information about what to use and what to watch out for, while the parents remain clear about the goals for their child and promptly report any changes, good or bad, they may notice.

Immediate and Long-Term Consequences

What we don't know about the effects of psychiatric drugs on the developing young brain and the impact on our children's future would fill far more books than what we do know. We are just beginning to acquire the tools that enable us to explore what occurs in the brain during development, and studies already show that profound changes in brain structure and organization continue at least into the early twenties. We have not even begun to explore how commonly used medications might affect those processes, for good or ill.

As a general rule, it seems that the effects of medications on young brains are immediate rather than long-lasting. Despite decades of using psychoactive medications, especially in older children and adolescents, no one has yet shown that they produce permanent changes in brain structure or function. (Little information,

even of this sort, is available for toddlers and preschoolers.) Although the absence of bad news is reassuring, it is quite possible we simply have not learned how or where to look. We have also not been able to discern whether medications actually might facilitate better brain development.

An Important Decision

If you've stayed with me this far, it should be clear that the decision to medicate your child is not a trivial one. You've probably asked questions like: "If the chosen drug doesn't work, do we try again?" "How many failures are too many?" "What if two, three, or even four drugs are needed to get the right benefits?" Some physicians urge, "Try it, you might like it. If not, you can always quit." But it can be hard to back off once you've decided to try medications. What if the next drug does what you were hoping for? On the other hand, if you have a child who is miserable and failing in key areas of development, how can you *not* try a drug that truly might make a difference?

The fact that you are reading this book is a sign of good parenting. If your child is not progressing in the ways you expected, you are absolutely right to look for more answers. The rest of this book shares guidelines I use in helping families think about this important decision.

Chapter 2

How to Find Professional Help

I have yet to meet a parent who came to see me on a whim. Seeking out the advice of a psychiatrist—or consulting another medical professional about a psychiatric disorder or behavior problem—generally happens only after a considerable period of time during which the parents tell themselves, or hear from others, such formulaic reassurances as: "The problem isn't all *that* bad," "It's just a phase; he'll grow out of it," "She's not really that different from other kids her age," or "I was just like him at that age."

Usually the final nudge toward seeking professional help comes from some outside source—a relative, a teacher, an article a parent has read, or a compelling television show. Often, these other sources put additional stress on the family. A preschool may suddenly decide that Jennifer isn't "ready" to be with other children. A soccer coach may suggest that Johnny simply doesn't fit in with the team. Other parents may stop letting their children come over to play. By the time parents seek help, most are con-cerned that something is wrong, but hopeful that "the expert" will find that they were worried for no reason.

Typically, the pediatrician is the first person to whom a family turns for help. Unfortunately, the average visit with a pediatrician now lasts about five minutes. While many families probably get satisfactory results from their pediatricians, those who eventually come to my office report the following responses from their doctors: "Let's wait and see; sometimes children are just slower to mature," or "Let's try putting little Harry on (insert medication of the day) and see if it helps."

Appropriately, parents are suspicious of both responses. They fear that a cursory diagnosis, no matter how experienced the eye, is inadequate. And they are absolutely right. Imagine coming to a doctor with complaints of chest pain and being told after only a few questions, "It's probably just gas—let's wait a few months to see if it gets better," or "Maybe it's a heart attack, so you better take these pills." Diagnosing childhood mental disorders is not often easy, and carefully targeted treatments are more likely to be safe and beneficial than those given without a reasonable understanding of the underlying problem.

As parents, you deserve (and should demand) the attention of a professional who has the skills and the time to carefully assess the situation. A doctor or mental health professional who is trained to work with children and adolescents should carefully analyze what is going on with your child and explore a reasonable range of possible solutions with you. If medication seems appropriate, the doctor should help you carefully monitor how your child is doing to be certain the medicine prescribed is the correct one.

One of the first and more obvious questions is how to find the right person to help you. This chapter will help you locate qualified professionals. It will also discuss how to determine if your child needs to be evaluated by a psychiatrist and the logistics of insurance companies and acquiring medication.

. . . .
When to Seek Help
. . . .

When a parent expresses concern about a child, physicians trained in looking for problems will be listening for some general red flags that might include the following types of behaviors:

- **Persistent**. As every parent knows, children go through phases. If there's a new baby in the family or if your child is starting kindergarten, it is not unusual for her to act out. Behavior that might be a cause for concern is behavior that persists. The problem may be constant or it may be recurring, gradually worsening with time.

- **Peculiar**. You will see a wide range of behaviors within your child's peer group —regardless of age. Yet, sometimes a child will exhibit behaviors that teachers and others who work with children find unusual. It may be simply a matter of timing; that is, a behavior may be appropriate in a younger child but not in a teenager. Other times, it is odd or bizarre behavior that warrants attention. For instance, four-year-olds often have imaginary friends they talk to; ten-year-olds generally do not.

- **Perturbing**. Disruptive behaviors can send warning signals from several different angles. If a child is disruptive within a classroom or a playgroup, you will likely be hearing directly from the teacher or group coordinator. But a child's behaviors may also be disruptive to himself. The sad and withdrawn child may not be very troublesome in class, but the behavior will keep the child from thriving and growing in the same way as his classmates. If your child's life is disrupted or not normal because of a concerning behavior, then it's important to get a professional opinion.

Overcoming Hesitations

Sometimes parents are so nervous about coming to see me that they procrastinate about making an appointment. They worry that by scheduling a session with a psychiatrist, they are somehow admitting there is something wrong with their child, or maybe even with themselves as parents. Nothing could be further from the truth. Think how wonderful you'll feel if you book an appointment, talk to a professional, and learn that there is no reason to worry. And, if there is cause for concern, you've taken the first step toward getting the help your child needs.

Although each chapter in Part Two describes various disorders and the associated symptoms, there are some commonly recognized behaviors that might lead you to ask your pediatrician about getting additional help. Remember, context is important. A single episode with a clear cause can probably be ignored; a major tantrum on the night before a household move, for example, is totally understandable.

The following list of symptoms is partially drawn from the Web site of the American Academy of Child & Adolescent Psychiatry (www.aacap.org).

Keep in mind that these are guidelines— even perfectly normal children and adolescents can occasionally show a few of these symptoms, especially when under stress. The key, again, is: persistent, peculiar, and perturbing.

Symptoms in Younger Children:
- Failure to keep up developmentally with peers (even children a year younger) in such expected milestones as language development, normal interest in toys and play, and peer friendships
- Worries or anxieties that seem excessive either in intensity or extent
- Excessive clinging and irritability that starts abruptly and without obvious cause
- Persistent nightmares
- Hyperactivity—fidgeting, constant movement beyond regular playing— that seem considerably greater than in peers
- Persistent disobedience or aggression
- Frequent temper tantrums
- Self-injurious behaviors, such as head banging or repeated biting of body parts (like arms or hands)
- Drop in school performance, especially if it previously was a source of pride

Symptoms in Preadolescents and Adolescents:
- Marked deterioration in school

performance, especially in children who previously were doing well

- Sudden, unexplained reduction in interest in a hobby or something formerly enjoyed—not just a change from one interest to another
- Recurrent inability to cope with problems that occur in daily life
- Persistent anger or irritability, or being overly emotional about many things
- Excessive preoccupation with something (such as making things very orderly) to the point that it is hard to do anything else
- Fear that seems excessive and pervasive
- Limited ability to concentrate or make decisions
- Unreasonable worry about doing something "bad"
- Need to wash, clean things, or perform certain routines dozens of times per day
- Definite and persistent changes in sleeping or eating patterns
- Numerous physical complaints, such as joint pains, stomachaches, or headaches without evidence of a medical illness
- Sustained or prolonged bad mood and attitude, often accompanied by poor appetite, difficulty sleeping, or a preoccupation with death
- Abuse of alcohol or drugs
- Intense fear of becoming obese, which bears no relationship to actual body weight, or purging or restrictive eating
- Threats of self-harm or harm to others, or actual self-injury or aggression
- Self-destructive behavior, such as cutting, burning, or repeated, deliberate, risky behaviors that could be dangerous; for example, opening the door of a moving car
- Repeated threats to run away or an actual attempt to do so
- Violations of the rights of others, such as opposing authority, truancy, thefts, or vandalism
- Strange thoughts or feelings and unusual behaviors, such as a fear of being poisoned or not wearing clothes someone else has touched
- Sexual behaviors that are inappropriate, excessive, or risky, such as multiple partners and repeated unprotected sex

Lists of this type can be helpful, but they tend to be either too broad or too narrow. I once had a patient whose mother, herself a highly qualified mental health professional, called me because her ten-year-old son had shaken her awake at 2 a.m. the night before and urgently told her to get up and put all the knives in the house somewhere safe because he was afraid he would lose control and use one to kill her. After telling me this, her first question was, "Is that normal?"

When I was in training, I became concerned about our second son, who was about ten months old, because he often seemed to avoid eye contact with both his mother and me. After vacillating between telling myself it was nothing and worrying it might be an early sign of some serious problem, I finally consulted a trusted colleague. My colleague helped me understand that our son was somewhat easily overstimulated and had trouble dealing with the noise his older brother tended to bring to the household. Sure enough, he was fine when we got him by himself. I realized I could stop worrying—at least about that.

Who to Consult

If some of the previous symptoms match your child's behavior, or if you are concerned about some other issue, consult with someone you know and trust who has some professional training—a school counselor or your child's pediatrician. Let them know in advance that you are concerned about your child's behavior and need advice. It may be best to meet first without your child so you can talk openly about the problem and plan a strategy for assessing it.

In order to have the full attention of the teacher, school psychologist, or pediatrician, call ahead to book an appointment. Schedule a time when you feel that person can best focus on your meeting. Schools and pediatricians' offices have several things in common, one of the primary ones being chaos at certain times of day and on certain days of the week. Monday mornings and Friday afternoons are notoriously busy in pediatric practices and in schools as well.

Worrisome behaviors are ones that are ongoing or have started abruptly with no recognizable cause. The history of when and how the behavior manifests itself should be part of your discussion with the professional. A parent is the best historian, particularly with younger children. The more you can organize your thoughts and observations in advance (in writing if possible), the clearer your presentation will be.

There are different ways to present your concerns. Narratives, where a parent describes in his or her own words specific events or a summary of events with recurrent themes, can be helpful. For example, you might tell the story of your daughter's tantrums that occur every time she doesn't get her way. Other parents are more detail-oriented, and for them a behavior diary may be highly useful. This is something you can keep in a journal or on your computer, or even note on a daily calendar.

However you decide to record the information, try to evaluate what might be most relevant. Besides the basic report of what happened, what you did about it, and how long it lasted, you might also want to note the time of day, the child's apparent mood before and after the event, and any unusual circumstances that may have had an influence, such as a particular food or being in a new place. Did anything change in your child's life around the time the behavior occurred—maybe a move, a new baby, or puberty? Have other family members had similar problems? If it is an unusual behavior (especially one that only occurs occasionally), consider videotaping it, as long as it doesn't upset the child. Don't worry too much about neatness or even completeness. The purpose is to keep the details fresh for when you review them later.

The more specific you can be about your concerns (providing examples where possible), the better prepared the professional will be to offer meaningful advice. If feasible, keep the originals and bring copies of your observations to the consultations. Most physicians and mental health specialists will have the capacity to copy papers and even videotapes, but it will take time that might be better spent gathering new information. Also, although it's rare, accidents do happen. A colleague once showed me a powerful video of temper outbursts of a young man who had previously been a patient. I asked him to make a copy of it for teaching pur-

poses and, because of a mix-up in the process, that precious tape was destroyed.

Do not be surprised if your first consultation fails to provide clear answers to your questions. Pediatricians and teachers are generalists, familiar with a broad range of problems but not necessarily experts at behavioral disorders. Good ones will be able to tell you if they have seen similar kinds of problems before, and whether they have the expertise to help. If they don't, they should be able to suggest referrals. If you feel that the answer they give is too generic, fails to fit your child, or simply does not address the concerns you have, insist on a referral.

Getting Referrals

Most pediatricians are under such strong time constraints these days that their ability to offer a variety of treatment interventions for mental disorders can be limited. Some will just prescribe medications, especially stimulants for ADHD and possibly antidepressants for depression or anxiety. As comfortable as it may feel to stay with the doctor who cared for your child from infancy, serious behavioral problems usually require the additional expertise and extra time a specialist can provide. Many pediatric practices are too busy overseeing the general health of growing children to carefully screen for a variety of issues (and some children may have several related issues) and carefully monitor the medications of a child who is having difficulty.

Americans believe that personal style and listening skills are the most important qualities for a mental health professional, according to a Therapy in America 2004 poll conducted by Harris Interactive. However, the survey revealed that three more practical factors usually determine how people actually choose this type of professional: physician recommendation, geographic location, and, increasingly, health plan coverage.

While having someone who listens to you and engenders your trust has indisputable merit, these factors aren't a bad way to get started:

Physician referral: Although your child's pediatrician may not have time to carefully consider some of the personal qualities you might like to have in a psychiatrist, psychologist, or social worker, the very fact that the referral comes from a professional enhances the likelihood that you'll see someone who has a good reputation and very likely has experience with the issue at hand. In this regard, a referral from a teacher, a principal, or a school psychologist can also be quite good, as they will be familiar with how these experts perform with children.

Geographic location: Families are pressed for time. For that reason, there is absolutely nothing wrong with starting out with the person who is most convenient geographically. If it works—and particularly if regular visits are necessary—this convenience will make life much less stressful. If teenagers are involved, selecting someone who is nearby can greatly increase your chance that they will continue to see the person. If it turns out that you don't like this person, you can always move on.

In-Network referral: If your medical care requires that you go to someone within your network, don't worry. Even if the person isn't the same ADHD specialist you've heard about from "everyone," this person sees many patients with similar problems within your health insurance network, and he or she will probably be fine. The peace of mind you gain by not having to worry about how you will pay for the evaluation is definitely a positive value. Also, if you find that all the identified providers are too busy to see you, you can turn to the insurance company to find someone else. That's their job.

Questions to Pose

Most medical practices are very busy, and

I'm well aware that our culture is not one that makes it easy for a patient to question a doctor about his or her background. However, you do want to feel comfortable with the medical professional you plan to see. In my opinion, running through a lengthy list of questions about qualifications is seldom productive; you can often get that type of information from wall plaques in their office, information posted on the Internet about the medical practice, or a biography on the Web site of the hospital with which the professional is affiliated. **If you are still uncertain, some useful questions are:**

- What proportion of your practice is with children the same age as my child?
- How long have you been practicing in this specialty?
- What do you do to make a child feel comfortable here?
- How do you assess children with problems like those my child has?
- What can my child and I expect during assessment and treatment, and how will we know if we're doing the right thing?

Adequate training is important, but so is empathetic listening, a style that fits with your own, and an openness to multiple possibilities, especially early on. Primarily, though, you want to observe how you and your child react to this professional. Compassion, concern, and a pleasant attitude toward the family are not enough to stand alone as qualifications, but they nicely complement competence.

If you are speaking to the professional at a pre-evaluation session, then it's easy to bow out if you get a bad feeling. If you're with your child, proceed with what you've committed to pay for. If the situation doesn't get better, or if the answers you receive fail to give you a better sense of what is happening to your child, don't be afraid to express your concern and reassess your options. Any reasonable professional will understand your concerns and will neither be threatened nor offended by such worries. The key is finding someone who will be your partner in helping your child. He or she doesn't have to be someone you'd like to invite for dinner, but mutual respect and shared concern for your child will be a big help in working together.

Insurance: Mental Health Care Coverage

Because you may be entering into a diagnosis and treatment process that may involve a good number of visits over a period of time, it is important that you investigate your insurance plan. The last thing you (or your child) needs is for you to suffer unnecessary stress over the bills.

TYPES OF PRACTITIONERS

There are many types of professionals you could encounter in pursuit of help for your child. Here's a brief rundown:

Child or Adolescent Psychiatrists must complete medical school, training in general psychiatry, and two additional years of advanced training before they can specialize in mental disorders of children and adolescents. All psychiatrists must be licensed as physicians by the state in which they practice. Child and adolescent psychiatrists are specialists in diagnosing and treating mental illnesses and can prescribe and monitor the use of psychoactive medications. They are also experts in other types of interventions, such as individual therapy, parent education, and family counseling.

Behavioral and Developmental Pediatricians take additional training after medical school and study general pediatrics to learn more about severe behavior problems, especially those that involve the body, such as bedwetting, problems with bowel control, eating disorders, learning problems, or behavior problems that arise from physical causes such as seizures.

Psychologists can earn doctoral degrees in clinical, educational, counseling, or research psychology. There is no formal specialty called "child psychology," but individuals can choose to obtain their training with younger populations. Psychologists can provide psychological testing and assessments and various forms of therapy for emotional and behavioral problems and disorders. They cannot prescribe medications, but may work with psychiatrists who can. Most states require psychologists to be licensed. Within the broad range of psychology are some subspecialties that may be of particular value for your child, such as educational psychologists or neuropsychologists.

Typical Plans

Insurance benefits for mental health and substance abuse differ among plans, employers, and states. In general, mental health coverage is not as good as regular medical coverage and may require higher deductibles and co-payments in addition to any regular fixed payments. Unfortunately, mental health coverage for children is almost always far less adequate than for adults.

The types of services insurance companies will pay for varies. In many parts of the country, for example, educational testing has now become the responsibility of

Clinical Social Workers have a master's degree in social work and can provide services for the prevention, diagnosis, and treatment of mental and behavioral disorders. They cannot prescribe medications, but they can refer patients to psychiatrists who can when appropriate. In most states, social workers take an examination to be licensed as clinical social workers.

Marriage and Family Therapists earn a certificate for training in counseling. Many work with children as well as with parents and families. They cannot prescribe medications; some work closely with physicians, others have independent practices. Most states have a licensing procedure.

Physician Assistants and Nurse Practitioners have advanced degrees and have received additional medical training. Some are licensed to prescribe medications, although usually in conjunction with a physician. Their level of independence varies from state to state, but they generally work within a medical office to manage patient care and are involved primarily in ongoing care rather than in diagnosis and initial care planning. Some, though still relatively few, have specialized training in mental illness or substance abuse; few specialize in working with children, let alone childhood psychiatric disorders.

If you've asked around for referrals and have not received any productive leads, the American Academy of Child & Adolescent Psychiatrists has an online referral directory (www.aacap.org). Enter your city and any requests as to specialty, and the directory will provide you with names. Of course, without a personal referral, you will want to double check that their practice is appropriate for your child.

---

the schools, not part of mental health coverage. On the other hand, legislation in many states has increased the responsibility of insurance companies to pay for treatment of a variety of behavioral disorders that were previously excluded from coverage. In 1996, the U.S. Congress passed the Mental Health Parity Act, with the intent of placing mental health benefits on par with other types of medical and surgical coverage. To date, however, the reality has fallen far short of the ideal in most parts of the country.

Most professionals will discuss these matters with you in advance. If they do not, bring the issue up yourself. You—and, for that matter, your mental health care provider—may have to be insistent (and persistent) to learn what is and is not covered. There are so many different kinds of plans that your doctor is unlikely to be able to fill in specifics on the spot, but he or she will be able to refer you to someone who can help you.

When you call your insurance plan or your company's benefits administrator, ask for a verbal and written description of what coverage is provided for mental health treatments or behavioral interventions—terms may vary. Especially important are matters of annual or lifetime caps for mental health benefits; that is, limits for each year or for total expenditures, after which all coverage ends. The American Academy of Child & Adolescent Psychiatry recommends you ask some of the following questions:

- Do I need a referral from my child's primary care physician or employee assistance program to receive mental health services?

- Is there a preferred list of providers or networks that we must see? Are there any child psychiatrists on this list? What happens if none of the approved providers can see us or if my child needs to see someone outside the network?

- Is there an annual deductible I must pay before the plan pays? What will I actually be charged for services? What services are covered by the plan: office visits, medication, respite care, day hospital, inpatient?

- Are there limits on the number of visits? Will my provider have to send reports to the managed care company?

- What can I do if I am unhappy with the care provider?

- What hospitals are covered under the plan?

- Does the plan exclude certain diagnoses or preexisting conditions?

AN IMPERFECT SYSTEM

One of my more painful memories is of an eight-year-old boy we were trying to hospitalize because he had spent almost all his waking hours for the previous week screaming at the top of his lungs. His insurance providers had a list of behavioral disorders not covered in their plan, but refused to tell either his parents or me what disorders were on that list. If we hospitalized him for a disorder not on the list, the insurance would pay the costs; otherwise, his parents would be fully responsible. Current regulations make such an impasse far less likely, but it still is worthwhile knowing ahead of time what is possible and what is not.

- Is there a "lifetime dollar limit" or an "annual limit" for mental health coverage, and, if so, what is it?
- Does the plan cover prescription medications?

Managed Care Plan

If you are a part of a managed care plan, then your insurance company may hire a subcontracted agent or take responsibility for overseeing your review. You may be assigned a case manager or utilization reviewer (generally a social worker or a nurse) who is responsible for monitoring your child's care, and the treating physician may need to discuss his or her plan with the case manager to be sure that it will be paid for by the insurance company. These reviews often take place over the telephone, but sometimes written plans are required. Some managed care plans want to see full medical records before authorizing treatment; others may authorize payment for a specific number of sessions. Managed care generally emphasizes short-term treatment with a focus on changing specific behaviors.

Preferred Provider Plan

If you're in a preferred provider plan, then you may have an arrangement where the insurance company will pay as long as you see someone in-network. If, for some reason, you choose to see a doc-tor outside the list (an "out-of-network" provider), your insurance company may not pay for the services or they may pay a much smaller share of the cost. Some hospitals are also considered out-of-network, so treatment there may not be covered. Even with preferred provider plans, some types of care may need to be discussed with a case manager, or there may be a referral requirement, whereby your child's pediatrician must make a referral in order for the visit to the specialist to be covered.

Employee Assistance Programs

Some employers offer employee assistance programs (EAPs). This resource is generally for company employees and their families for substance abuse, stress, depression, and other mental health issues. The programs generally offer preventive care such as health screenings, mental health or substance abuse screenings, and wellness activities. This program is often free, but the number of visits may be limited. These EAP visits are totally confidential, and no information from them is ever shared with an employer.

You may also decide to see someone out of your plan and pay the fee directly. Be aware, however, that many insurance plans will not only refuse to pay for those visits but also for any tests or medications recommended, as well as more expensive interventions such as hospitalization or day treatment. Discuss such possibilities fully with that individual and your insurance representative before proceeding on a course that may be unacceptably costly.

Medical Savings Accounts

If you are eligible, tax-exempt contributions to medical savings accounts (MSAs) can help pay medical expenses until your insurance plan kicks in. People who work for companies with fewer than fifty employees and have a high deductible or employee-sponsored health plan are generally eligible for an MSA. This account can be used to supplement your health insurance plan if your deductible is above $1,500 or more annually per individual, or $3,200 or more per family. In addition to MSA contributions being tax-exempt, families get to keep any unspent money in the account, so you are not penalized for putting money away for a medical "rainy day."

Similar to MSAs, some companies offer flexible spending accounts, which can also be used to supplement costs for items not covered by your insurance. The rules on these are tighter, so check on the rules that govern your company's plan before signing up for one.

The Cost of Medication

If your child needs medications, it can be costly. Many do not have a generic (and less expensive) form, and the prices for name-brand medications reflect research and development costs (it takes three to five years to study a new drug, and another four or five to test it). The range can go from twenty to several hundred dollars per month.

Obviously, you don't want to pay for a medicine that turns out to be ineffective, so ask your doctor for free samples or a small initial supply if possible. Then, if the medication proves effective, investigate the least expensive way to order it. (For example, your insurance plan may want you to use a three-month-supply mail-order system.) If a generic version is available, check with the prescribing physician to see if it is equally as effective as the brand-name medication.

Sometimes, plans will only cover medications recommended by your primary care physician. If this is the case, most doctors are quite willing to rewrite the prescription of a medication recommended by a specialist. Be sure to also confirm that your insurance will pay for your child's specific medications. Occasionally, insurance plans will pay for one type of medication within a class (such as antidepressants), but not another. Let your doctor know if this occurs. It is usually fine to switch, but not always. Special procedures exist for these kinds of situations, so getting the medication your child needs may simply entail additional paperwork.

Other cost-saving methods include buying in bulk or asking for a prescription of a higher dosage and then splitting the pill. If you opt for this method, double-check with the prescribing physician to be certain that splitting the pill doesn't affect the integrity of the medication. If the pill can be split safely, then do so the moment the prescription enters your house.

People often take too much medication because they don't pay attention to dosage strength.

For families with low incomes, all U.S. pharmaceutical companies have compassionate-care programs to provide necessary medications. However, most of these programs require you to exhaust all other options first; to qualify you will need to provide proof of income as well as support from your prescribing doctor.

What You Can Do in the Meantime

The families I see are in pain. They are

worried about their children, they are worried about what is happening, and they are concerned that they may have done something wrong. If you were in my office, I would do what I could to alleviate your worries. I would remind you that looking for help for your child is a sign of good parenting; no matter what answers you get, you can rest assured that you are doing the right thing simply by investigating the issue.

Between now and the time you get a formal diagnosis and treatment plan, families should remember that the child is suffering, and there are a couple of things you can do to help:

- **Catch them being good.** The four-year-old who simply won't sit down, the eight-year-old who cries frequently or dawdles constantly, and the fourteen-year-old who often acts out in class are all children who do not get much positive feedback, and families sometimes get caught up in a yelling/blaming cycle. Start making a big effort to notice the good things and comment on them. It may be difficult to find the moment when a four-year-old slows down enough to compliment him on gently petting the dog or bringing his lunch dish to the kitchen, but compliments do wonders at building self-esteem.
- **Don't blame.** Parenting 101 says that you should criticize the behavior but

not the child. "Don't throw those toys" is psychologically very different from saying, "Bad kids throw toys." If you feel your entire relationship is built on scolding, take a step back and correct only the dangerous behaviors; try to ignore and move beyond the annoying ones until you've begun to better communicate how much you love your child.

- **Plan something fun to do together.** Think of an activity your child would enjoy that is not stressful. (Taking a rambunctious first-grader to see a ballet would be stressful—for everyone!) At first, fifteen minutes of a pleasant activity may be the best that can be achieved. The more frequently you spend pleasurable time together, the easier it will be to help your child overcome any behavioral issues.
- **Don't give up.** Keep an open mind, because sometimes problems truly do go away on their own. However, in the vast majority of cases I have seen, persistence has been crucial. If you cannot see "the expert" as quickly as you want, consider accepting the referral to a colleague or making an appointment for a later date. You can always cancel if you find the help you need before then.

Sometimes finding a professional you trust who understands your child and can work with you is easy. Much more often, it takes time, persistence, and initiative on your part. My best advice is to beware of extremes. If someone promises you, sight unseen, that he's seen thousands of children just like yours and knows exactly what you need—which just happens to be what he offers—it probably is too good to be true. If a friend, teacher, or even your pediatrician tells you that the only person who can help you is Dr. So-and-So, that's also highly unlikely. If you have several promising leads and one is available before another, it's reasonable to start there.

However, don't engage in parallel evaluations (i.e., seeing more than one specialist for the same issue for comparison purposes). It's costly, more likely to be confusing rather than helpful, and an additional strain on health care systems that are already overtaxed.

Most of all, have faith in yourself and your family. You are the genuine expert on your child. What you are looking for is someone to be your ally while providing you with additional knowledge about your child's problem.

Chapter 3

How Diagnoses Are Made

"Why have you come to see me?" is one of the first questions I ask when I meet a new family. It seems like such a simple question, but it elicits a great deal of helpful information. If possible, I also like to pose some variation of that question to each family member—and I often get very different answers from each person. Common responses from children range from "I don't know" to "Because I'm bad." They'll also mention a range of symptoms, such as not paying attention, hitting others, or "being mad all the time." Similarly, parents' responses vary considerably.

A surprising number of families are truly baffled at finding themselves in my office. Many times, they are there because someone—a teacher, a judge, a pediatrician—sent them to me to "fix" their child; such families are often suspicious of me and, at least initially, resistant to the evaluation process. Others are absolutely certain they know what the problem is. A teacher or family friend may suspect the child has a specific disorder; and indeed,

when the parents researched that diagnosis on the Internet, they agreed. Such families often arrive in my office with a checklist that proves this theory about their child. They have little interest in wasting my time and their money confirming what they already know; they just want a medication or plan to solve the problem.

Unfortunately, the answer is rarely that simple. Making an accurate diagnosis of a psychiatric disorder in a child or adolescent typically requires a good amount of time by a qualified and dedicated practitioner. There is no blood test, EKG, or fancy probe for mental disorders. What is required is someone who can take the time to do a detailed evaluation and really look at all the pieces of the puzzle. A divorce, a new sibling, or the trauma of a cross-country move can all exacerbate a child's behavior to the point that it seems disordered, but only a trained professional will know how to evaluate whether the behavior is something that will be resolved on its own (postdivorce, post-baby, post-move, etc.) or whether there is something else going on.

Why Pediatricians Don't Usually Diagnose

Comprehensive evaluations take time. The typical pediatrician has between five and ten minutes to decide on a rough diagnosis and plan for the next step, whether it be further diagnostic procedures or treatment. Imagine a rambunctious seven-year-old who is trying to dismantle every available piece of equipment in a doctor's office as the mother describes how he terrorizes all the other kids in his class. An experienced pediatrician is apt to suspect ADHD and may well recommend a trial of medication. He might even suggest, "Well, let's try him on a little Ritalin; then we'll know if it's ADHD." He then writes out the prescription, gives a few instructions for taking it, and schedules a routine follow-up appointment for a month later.

Unfortunately, this well-meaning doctor could quite possibly be doing the child and the family a terrible disservice. It is entirely possible that the child has a multilayered problem that only looks like ADHD, or of which ADHD is only a part. Equally important is the close and careful monitoring of the medication's effects, especially in the beginning. No one pill and dosage is right for all children, so families need to see a professional who can continually evaluate whether or not the right medication and correct dosage is being given.

Getting a proper diagnosis requires much more than simply identifying and counting up symptoms. Some years ago, I met with Simon, who was almost nine years old and had received an ADHD diagnosis about a year earlier. Simon's parents brought him to see me because he was taking 180 mg of Ritalin a day (more than three times the recommended daily amount) with little apparent benefit, and no notable side effects. They were not aware that he was on an exceptionally high dose, just that his "ADHD" was not responding to medication.

I found it very interesting that the parents were clear that Simon's problems developed abruptly, shortly after his eighth birthday. Even when pushed, they recalled no real concerns about attention, impulsivity, or hyperactivity before then, either at home or at school. Rather, he seemed to just "fall apart," becoming more irresponsible at home and at school, not following orders the way he used to, making messes at home and not cleaning them up unless told to do so, and being more "scatterbrained." A teacher suggested ADHD, and a brief visit to the pediatrician got them their first Ritalin prescription. A small dose seemed to have helped. Although the parents could not exactly say what got better, they did recall that the benefit wore off after a week or so, His dose was increased, but again the benefit wore off after a short time. Simon underwent multiple dosage increases, each increase restoring the benefit briefly.

Many aspects of this story failed to ring true to me as a description of ADHD. It is not a disorder that suddenly appears at age eight, nor is it one for which medication's effects repeatedly wear off over such a short time span. Also, as his parents described their frustrations with Simon, it became clear that their major complaint had to do with his being irresponsible; he had few, if any, clear symptoms of inattention, let alone impulsivity or hyperactivity.

As we reviewed Simon's history in more detail, I learned that the parents had adopted Simon a few months after he was born. They knew little about his biological parents, other than that his mother was in her late teens and reportedly had not abused medications, at least while pregnant. He seemed developmentally healthy and had at least normal intelligence with no evidence of learning disabilities.

It turned out that shortly before Simon began having problems, his adoptive mother, who had been home full-time, had to take a job because of financial pressures. That meant that Simon's parents expected him to help out more around the home and be more independent and self-reliant. To his parents' intense frustration, the more they

expected of him, the less reliable he became.

After several sessions alone with Simon, I learned that he felt his parents had become less available and more critical. Knowing that he had already been "rejected" by his biological mother, he thought that this was a prelude to the same thing with his adoptive parents. Simon feared that by meeting their demands to be more independent he was hastening the time when he'd be sent away again.

We got Simon off his Ritalin, which he did not need, and worked with him and his family to clarify their miscommunication. They were horrified to learn that he could believe them capable of sending him away, and we had to work on their guilt as well as his suspiciousness. Simon also needed to talk with a counselor about his feelings of rejection by his biological mother. As the family started to become more comfortable with each other again, all of Simon's "ADHD" symptoms evaporated.

An Accurate Diagnosis

An accurate diagnosis should take into consideration a wide range of factors—meaning that the professional should be aware that some issues may overlap traditional boundaries. One well-accepted framework for collecting this information is called the biopsychosocial model. It challenges the psychiatrist to consider

BE WARY OF "QUICK AND EASY"

Unfortunately, in matters of the brain and behavior, there are no shortcuts. In my part of the country, there is an aggressive group (with offices nationwide) that advertises for brain imaging (SPECT scans). Its ads proclaim that imaging is a "definitive diagnostic tool" for identifying a variety of severe mental disorders, including ADHD, depression, OCD, and anxiety, as well as clarifying the causes of problem behaviors such as violence.

I am reminded of a patient I saw recently. A school counselor had recommended the brain imaging clinic because Mason, a seventeen-year-old junior in high school, was not doing as well academically as he and his parents wanted; otherwise, he was fine. The parents paid $5,000 for their son to be evaluated, the major cost being for two brain scans. Afterward, the doctor sat down with Mason's mother and wrote prescriptions for four different medications—Mason had never taken psychiatric medication before. (For me, it takes an extraordinary situation to write a prescription for more than one medication at a time. You never know how someone is going to react to medications, so trying them out one at a time is essential.) The mother had finally had enough when the doctor explained that the fourth medication was for Mason's "violent behaviors." When she protested that he had never, ever, been violent, the doctor pointed to one of the scans and said, "See, it shows up right here." Ultimately, this family realized that they had paid $5,000 they could ill afford, only to then need to look elsewhere for a less technologically sophisticated, but far more useful, evaluation. This new evaluation revealed that the family's instincts were correct: Mason simply had some problems with inattention and had not learned how to study or allocate his time optimally.

There may be other clinics or centers in your area that promise alternative diagnostic methods or herbal cures, or may claim your child's problem is caused by allergies. (Sometimes their ads are so appealing and promise such wonderful results that I'm tempted to go to them myself!) Unfortunately, there are no shortcuts. You need someone who will not only assess what is wrong but also monitor treatment. Don't try to cut corners with this process.

---

biological factors, such as genetics, physical development, and physical diseases; *psychological* factors, such as the child's mood states, specific behaviors, attitudes, and experiences; and *social* factors, such as family issues, parenting styles, economic status, and major life events. Past events are often as important as current ones, especially as they reveal the course of a child's problems over time. Development is also a key point to consider with children and adolescents. What should one expect of a child at this age? How different is that from what is happening?

Buttressing this sometimes daunting accumulation of information may be formal testing, which provides information about intellectual function and specific strengths and weaknesses in the brain. It can also offer insights into how a child handles information and emotional situations. Most of this testing is done by psychologists and assesses performance on standardized tests and physical manipulation of objects; that is, having the child answer questions on a range of topics and perform tasks that include solving puzzles and sorting shapes. There are also neurological procedures such as the EEG (electroencephalogram), the MRI (magnetic resonance imaging), or other brain scans. However, unless there is reason to suspect a child might be prone to seizures or have a brain tumor (almost always accompanied by changes in physical function), such expensive interventions don't provide information that will help enhance diagnostic precision or inform treatment recommendations. There is some fascinating research that uses these tests to study how brains of individuals with ADHD, autism, bipolar disorder, and other psychiatric disorders diverge from normal brains, but none are ready for clinical applications.

A biopsychosocial assessment can reveal not only one or more diagnoses, but also the "story" of a family and child. This story, called a formulation, organizes information and brings together the various threads into a coherent whole. It puts diagnoses in a more proper and complete context, and can often suggest what interventions are most likely to be beneficial.

GETTING THE BEST EVALUATION

The best evaluations occur when all parents or guardians are involved. If work schedules or divorce make it difficult for one or both parents to attend the sessions regularly, the absent parent should still try to stop in as often as possible—he or she may be able to provide useful insight into the situation. Sometimes I request that the whole family come in together, so I can see how family members interact, both positively and negatively. Otherwise, I suggest that parents with two or more children bring only the identified patient. The best outcome for the child will come if everyone is given the opportunity to focus completely on that child. Having to divert one's attention in order to keep an anxious or bored brother or sister from disrupting the process is not the best way for a parent to help their child.

Keeping Secrets and Confidentiality

There are many reasons why, but sometimes parents hold back relevant information. This is understandable, but not helpful. A physician's diagnosis is only as good as the information on which he or she bases it. The fact that a ten-year-old is still sleeping with the parents is information relevant to a diagnosis. If parents are seriously contemplating a divorce but are avoiding telling anyone "to protect the family," their tension with each other may be part of their child's problem. A mother whose own mother committed suicide may hesitate to reveal that fact to her suicidal daughter, lest she "sends her over the edge." It almost certainly won't, but the hidden fear will surely affect the mother's ability to help her child. Revealing past or ongoing sexual abuse will be disruptive to the family, but keeping it secret in hopes that it will just go away cripples any reasonable assessment.

One common reason for keeping secrets is the parents' fear that they will be blamed. Indeed, early practitioners of psychiatry took the view that parents— especially mothers—were guilty until proven innocent. Now, however, it is clear that most of the time no one person or thing causes a disorder. It just happens. It wasn't that one glass of wine during preg-nancy or the vaccine your child was given at age two. It wasn't that you were too strict or not strict enough. Nevertheless, knowledge of those aspects of a child's history can help to both clear the air and contribute to changes can be made.

During evaluations, I agree not to violate either the child's or the parents' confidentiality—although I almost always urge them to get relevant information out in the open as quickly and appropriately as possible. Still, there are important exceptions to confidentiality that everyone needs to understand from the outset. Professionals are required by law to take action when someone makes a serious threat of suicide or homicide; similarly, any description of behaviors that suggest a child or adolescent has been or is being exposed to sexual or physical abuse or to severe neglect must be reported to the appropriate authorities.

To someone harboring a secret like abuse, it must be almost impossible to imagine what the world will be like once the secret is out. Many families assume that the mere mention of such an issue inevitably derails an assessment. Nothing is further from the truth. Yes, part of my job is to ensure that appropriate authorities are informed when someone is in danger, but the rest of my job is to help support families through such a crisis and to continue to explore what is happening and what to do about it. I have the parents help me file an official report if necessary, explaining to them and the child what will happen. Once others have taken responsibility for dealing with that aspect of the problem, we can continue looking at the broader issues, including how the abuse or other reportable matter may have contributed to the family's decision to come see me.

Except for the specific topics just mentioned, mental health professionals are under strict regulations to protect your confidentiality. For example, you may have decided to come see me because of a recommendation from your best friend whose son I treated. However, even though the two of you can talk about me all you want, I am not supposed to admit to even knowing your friend and her child unless I have explicit written permission from them to discuss their care with you. Similarly, you have the power to decide who I can contact to gather information or share findings about your child.

One other major exception to this rule of confidentiality is the insurance company paying the bills. The federal Health Insurance Portability and Accountability Act of 1996 (HIPAA), in the guise of tightening confidentiality for the individual, also guaranteed that insurance companies can have access to and share with each other any information they need to determine the appropriateness of bills submit-

ted to them. Such sharing of information is highly unlikely to create a problem for you or your child, but you cannot withhold information from the insurance company if they are being asked to pay for any portion of the cost.

The Process

Frequently, parents are dismayed that all I do is "just talk" with them. For better or for worse, however, that's where most of the raw data a psychiatrist needs comes from. I want to meet with the family together, with the child separately, and with the parents separate from the child. The order varies, depending on the age of the child and type of problem, but the general pattern is the same.

A psychiatrist will usually ask for information about the following:

- Description of the present problems and symptoms
- General health, illness, and treatments (both physical and psychiatric), including current medications
- The child's development
- School and friends
- Family relationships
- Parent and family health and psychiatric histories
- How the parents were raised
- Major trauma or other stressors for the

child and family, past or present

- Psychiatric interview of the child
- If necessary, laboratory studies such as blood tests, X-rays, or special assessments (for example, psychological, educational, hearing, speech, or language evaluation)
- With parents' permission, information from other significant people, such as family physician, school personnel, or other relatives

Some professionals standardize their collection of background information by asking the family to fill out a multipage form before their first visit. Typically, such a form includes sections on family history of illness, information about other family members, questions about birth history and early development, and details about schooling. A variety of standardized questionnaires are also available that cover either broad areas of behavioral disturbances or specific sets of symptoms associated with a particular disorder. These forms can be especially useful in gathering information from nonfamily members who deal with the child outside the home. These questionnaires are meant to identify the presence or absence of symptoms, but are not designed to give diagnoses.

The Initial Consultation

When possible, I like to start my first session with a new patient by meeting with everyone say hello, talk a bit about why they have come to see me, and agree on a game plan. Sometimes, however, this is neither feasible nor appropriate. For example, an adolescent forced into coming will probably not want to sit and listen to his parents' litany of complaints, so I would probably first meet with him alone. Sometimes, divorced parents may not want to attend joint sessions, so I may meet with them separately. My purpose is to gather information, not cause further trauma.

When I meet with a family for the first time, I have two goals: To put the family at ease, and to find out why they have come to see me now. Unfortunately, there is still a lot of guilt and shame involved in consulting a psychiatrist. Parents worry that they could have done more, that they could have been "better parents." They ruminate on "if only. . ." scenarios. I try to convey to families that, in most cases, nothing they could have done would have changed things, and even if there was, the important job now is to figure out how to help their child. For the depressed teen, the ADHD child, or the toddler with autism, the key issue is seldom how it happened, but rather what we can do about it.

In addition to helping them relax, I also want to know why the family finally decided to see someone—what was the straw that broke the camel's back? These

ABOUT THE DSM

While pursuing solutions to your child's problem, you may hear reference to the *Diagnostic and Statistical Manual of Mental Disorders* (DSM). Now in its fourth edition—often called the DSM-IV—this book is essentially an encyclopedia of mental disorders. For each disorder, the DSM lists specific criteria for making a diagnosis and provides background information about commonality by gender, age, and ethnicity; how the diagnosis manifests over time; whether it runs in families; and what other diagnoses might look like it (called a differential diagnosis). It does not discuss treatment options. When the government and private insurers started paying for mental health services and tying reimbursement to specific diagnoses in the mid-1980s, the manual grew increasingly more important.

If you've ever read a magazine article about an illness or a mental disorder and suddenly "discovered" you have the illness because you seem to have a good number of the symptoms, then you'll understand the limitations of the DSM. If you were to sit down and read it, you might find several disorders from which you, your spouse, or your children appear to suffer. That's where professional expertise comes in. Many of the issues described as "symptoms" in the DSM can also be perfectly normal behavior in certain individuals.

One day, a professor and his son came to see me. The professor had been reading the DSM, and was convinced that both he and his twelve-year-old son had Asperger's disorder, a severe developmental disorder characterized by marked social delays and a range of odd preoccupations or unusual behaviors. After evaluating the child and speaking at length with the father about his own history, I explained why neither of them had the disorder. It was true that both of them were uncomfortable at social functions and were easily overwhelmed in large groups, but neither of them had trouble reading and sending nonverbal social cues, and both were able to form and maintain age-appropriate social connections with others. In addition, the only "odd" behavior the father could identify for himself was a love of numismatics (coin collecting), which was a long-standing hobby. His son loved to play video games more than his father would have preferred, but otherwise had no odd behaviors. He had friends and was doing well in school. In short, beyond the father's sense that "something must be wrong," there were no clear signs or symptoms of a disorder. In addition, there was no evidence that any of the behaviors the father identified in himself or his son were impairing their ability to function. There was only the father's concern, after reading a checklist of symptoms, that he was overlooking a serious problem.

problems tend not to sneak up on a family—chances are, they have been dealing with the situation for quite some time. What made the family decide to seek help now? How long have they been concerned? Typically, a family will have a long story about behaviors that have concerned them over time, but there is usually one final occurrence that put them over the edge. It could have been a warning from school or simply being at their wit's end in dealing with the child, but I want to know why the visit became important to them *now*.

During this first meeting, I pay particular attention to who speaks and who stays silent, as well as how people react to the information being presented. If anyone gets too uncomfortable I intervene, suggesting we can talk about sensitive issues at a later time. I directly ask silent family members how they see things, or if there is anything they want to add. I quickly step in if families start demonstrating some of the battles that go on at home, emphasizing that my purpose is to help, not to be a mediator.

Meeting with the Child

During the initial consultation process, I like to spend time alone with the child or adolescent, and will ask whether this needs to happen before or after I have spoken with the parents. Some children find it almost impossible to separate from their parents and may be unwilling to do so the first time we meet; others can't wait for them to leave so I can hear the "real story." These sessions can take place on the same day or can be spread out over several days or even weeks, depending on our schedules, the family's wishes, or insurance coverage.

My interview with the child has two general purposes. Partly, I want the child to tell me, in her own words, what is going on. Sometimes I may want to see or at least hear about a certain behavior, like a motor tic or a particular obsession. Mostly, though, I am content just to hear what the child has to say—or not say—about the situation. This is especially important with so-called "internalizing" disorders, such as anxiety and depression, because only the child knows his own thoughts and feelings. Many children are remarkably perceptive about their problems and how they might better avoid them. Many also carry their own load of guilt about why they are so "bad" or "mean" or "lazy," and I begin to give them the same message I want the parents to hear: Blame isn't the name of the game; making things better is. I emphasize to the child that what she tells me is just between us, except if she is thinking about hurting herself or someone else, or if someone else is hurting her. I assure her that, if there is something that someone else needs to know, we will discuss the matter and figure out what to do together. I also stress that the more I know about what's happening, the more likely it is I can help.

With adolescents, I usually do a talking-only interview. With young children, I may use toys or games as a way of making the child more comfortable, and also as an additional source of information. Often, when children tell their parents that we "just played," the parents worry that I have failed to see the "real problem." However, younger children have little ability to report on their on behaviors; I need to get that information in a different way. From the child, I am looking for different kinds of data. Can the child stay on task? Does he know the rules and follow them or make them up and change them? What kind of relationship does he try to develop with me? How does he handle transitions or sudden noises? What happens when the parents leave? When they come back?

When I meet with the parents alone, I cover much of the same ground. Parents are also better able to fill in important aspects of the child's or family's history. Do mental disorders run in the family, and if so, which ones? What, if anything, was going on when the problem first occurred? How have they tried to remedy the situation, and what were the results? What do they fear is going on? What have other professionals told them, and how did they react to those evaluations?

Gathering Additional Information

Depending on the questions being posed, I may decide that I need information beyond what the child and parents can provide. Common additional information includes:

Medical history. Information from the child's pediatrician or family health care practitioner, including any known medical problems, often provides a helpful additional perspective.

Information from the school. Insights about both academic performance and school behavior can be gained from questionnaires that focus on specific behavioral concerns, direct interviews with teachers by phone or in person, or a school visit to observe the child.

Cognitive testing. Part of the problem might relate to how the child thinks and learns, so formal cognitive testing from a qualified psychologist affiliated with the school may be beneficial. Such tests help clarify how a child takes in and processes information, and may identify certain areas of relative strength or weakness. They can be especially helpful in addressing questions of chronic poor performance at school.

Projective testing. Sometimes children are unable or unwilling to describe their thoughts. Psychologists have developed several tests that indirectly explore such questions by inviting children to talk about what they see in pictures or respond to open-ended questions. Although seldom diagnostic, these types of tests can offer valuable insights.

Medical evaluation. If there is reason to believe that a child's problem might have a physical cause (such as seizures or thyroid issues), additional medical work-ups may be advantageous. These studies are better coordinated through the pediatrician, as medical insurance coverage is almost always better than psychiatric coverage.

Sometimes videos can be enormously helpful, especially with behaviors that the family has trouble describing and are sure the physician will never see. In one in-stance, I was assessing a seven-year-old patient with symptoms of severe mental retardation and autism. According to his family, he had been fine until about three and a half years of age, when he changed abruptly. The father had created a detailed video history of their child from birth to the present, with many thirty- to sixty-second clips taken at different ages. In addition to documenting how normal he was early on, the family actually caught on tape the first time he fell apart—he broke down over a minor disappointment and became totally inconsolable. It was a fascinating, if heartbreaking, montage that proved very helpful in clarifying the diagnosis.

Another patient I saw for an autism evaluation was memorable for a different reason. He seemed to be a perfectly unre-markable eight-year-old, however, since

PAST EVALUATIONS

Some parents don't want me to know anything about testing or evaluations that have been done in the past. Usually, they are worried that I can't be objective after reading others' con-clusions. Such sentiments are especially common if the parents disagree with the previous diagnosis or if it puts them in a bad light. Although such concerns are easy enough to under-stand, I believe they are misplaced. The fact of the matter is that the other doctor is a trained professional who will have important, documented information about the child. I certainly en-courage parents to explain why they decided they didn't trust the doctor, feel he didn't spend enough time on analysis, or was dismissive of information they provided—but I am better able to do my job taking care of a child if parents share any and all professional reports.

the age of three, he reportedly could only watch TV while standing up and flapping both arms. At first, he refused to discuss this admittedly unusual behavior and was too shy to demonstrate it. Fortunately, his mother had captured his flapping on video. As he and I watched it together, I was able to assure him and his parents that this was in no way suggestive of autism; he just had an odd habit—a stereotypic movement disorder—that was not going to be a problem for him.

Explaining the Results

After you've spent so much time trying to be as clear as possible about what is happening to your child, what should you expect in return? There is no single answer. At the very least, you should get a reasonably accurate reflection of the information you provided, like the formulation, or story, mentioned earlier. Even if parts of that story are painful to hear, they should ring true as a faithful description of your child and your experience. From this should emerge a specific diagnosis, or at least a clear statement of probable causes for your child's difficulties. At this point, a treatment plan can start to take shape.

Many parents want to know what the future holds. That hinges on many factors, including the child's age, disorder, overall level of function, and response to treatment. Naturally, it is far easier to predict

how a seventeen- or eighteen-year-old will be as a young adult than it would be for a two-year-old. I usually talk about ranges of outcomes I've seen with similar children, emphasizing that only time will give us the real answer.

When it comes to providing families with a written diagnosis, professionals vary markedly. Psychologists who perform formal testing almost always provide a typed report, often quite lengthy, that details the test results, conclusions about those results, and recommendations. Physicians, including child and adolescent psychiatrists, may provide anything from verbal feedback to a handwritten note to a typed report. Be aware that many mental health professionals have little to no secretarial assistance, and report-generation is seldom covered by insurance. For example, I type up all my own reports (in part because it is true what they say about doctors' handwriting). If you need to have something in writing (e.g., as part of a school evaluation), make sure to let the professional know as quickly possible in order to avoid frustration and confusion.

Following Up

Offering a general guideline about follow-up is difficult because there are so many possibilities. You may be returning to your original caregiver, hopefully with new insights into your child's problems and specific suggestions about next steps. You may be continuing with the person who just finished the assessment, and moving from evaluation to treatment. You may have to find new providers of recommended services. If you are seeing someone strictly for a consultation, for example, your last contact may be the feedback session, with or without a formal written report. You may receive treatment referrals, and it is perfectly reasonable to discuss future contacts if questions or new problems arise. Quite often, the assessment phase leads directly into treatment with the same individual. For example, if your child has received a diagnosis of depression and antidepressants seem appropriate, the last part of the feedback session might include details about starting a medication and a return visit scheduled for a few days to a week later. I strongly recommend that you and the professional acknowledge explicitly that you are moving into a new phase of your work together, and discuss issues such as the frequency and cost of visits and standards for evaluating their value over time.

ATTENTION TO DETAIL

When I work with new medical students, I give them the following diagnostic exercise: "A mother phones you because she thinks her child has a problem: He refuses to pay attention, he doesn't follow commands, he's constantly getting out of his seat without permission." Then I ask these future doctors, "What's the next step in figuring out whether this child should be seen?" A good number of the students will immediately talk about assessing the child for other symptoms of ADHD, but usually at least one excellent clinician-in-the-making will say, "Wait. Do we know how old this child is?"

That's the kind of attitude and sensitivity you're looking for in a good diagnostician—someone who can take small bits of information and form a picture that helps you better understand your child's issue. In this example, the symptoms are age-appropriate for toddlers, but might suggest ADHD in an older child. You need someone who listens carefully and pays attention to the small clues that define your child's situation.

PART TWO

Understanding Behavioral and Mood Disorders

The following chapters will provide you with a better understanding of the symptoms and the nature of many common behavioral or mood disorders. Whether a teacher has said to you, "I think Jimmy must have ADHD," or a pediatrician has indicated that your child should be further evaluated for depression or some type of developmental delay, these chapters can help clarify the issues that can arise.

The next four chapters cover the four different types of behavioral and mood disorders, including:

- **Attention and disruptive behavior disorders** (attention-deficit/hyperactivity disorder, oppositional defiant disorder, and conduct disorder)
- **Affective disorders** (depression, dysthymic disorder, and bipolar mood disorder)
- **Anxiety-type disorders** (generalized anxiety disorder, separation anxiety, panic attacks, phobias, post-traumatic stress disorder, and sleeping problems)
- **Early developmental disorders** (mental retardation, autism, and Asperger's disorder)

Each disorder is discussed separately, with explanations broken into four sections: "What Is It?," "What Causes It?," "The Diagnosis," and "Treatment." Sometimes the discussions expand beyond these general topics; for example, there's a great deal to say about ADHD because now there is so much scientific information—but also because there are still so many misunderstandings about the disorder. Most of the descriptions also feature anecdotes that are composites of patients I've seen.

Treatments are covered more fully in other sections of the book (medications are discussed at length in Part Three, and non-drug therapies are discussed in Part Four). However, for each disorder I try to give some indication of suitable treatment options. After you've read this section, please turn to the appropriate parts of the book to read about treatments in more detail.

My intention is not to give you the tools with which to make your own diagnosis and treatment plan, but rather to ensure that you have sufficient knowledge about what is happening to your child and that you are an informed partner in the treatment process. I also want you to see that every child has a story, and every family has its challenges—even the brilliant or beautiful child can put a family through some uneasy times.

Chapter 4

Attention and Disruptive Behavior Disorders

Six-year-old Jerritt can't sit still in class, but at home he plays video games for hours without getting up; his ten-year-old sister, Rheanne, daydreams in school and at home and is easily bored. Twelve-year-old Tomas kicks the walls in the house, picks fights at school, and constantly uses foul language. Thirteen-year-old Rick routinely throws tantrums when he doesn't get his way, lies constantly, and has been disciplined for truancy several times.

All children misbehave sometimes, but with attention-deficit/hyperactivity disorder (ADHD) (Jerritt and Rheanne), oppositional defiant disorder (ODD) (Tomas), or conduct disorder (Rick), these behaviors are chronic and have a major effect on the lives of the children themselves and of those around them. This cluster of disorders, which frequently occur together in the same child, often are called disruptive or externalizing disorders. While children who have them can some-

times calm down and concentrate or behave, most of the time they are very much as the term implies: disruptive to themselves and to those around them.

If you are the parent of one of these children, or are close to someone who is, I scarcely need to tell you how difficult and exhausting they can be. When they are young, you worry constantly about the accidental or deliberate mischief they may be getting into; as they grow older, their capacity for wreaking havoc and irritating others simply keeps expanding. With the well-meaning child, as my own son was, you may grow weary of the countless times they sincerely apologize for breaking something, for forgetting to follow through on a task or assignment, or even just for not listening—again! With those children who are angry and deliberately hurtful, you repeatedly feel like a failure as a parent and cringe at the tongue-lashings you get from both your child and other adults who are more than willing to inform you of what a bad job you are doing. In a two-parent family, these children can place enormous strains on the marriage, because one parent may be more sympathetic about or intolerant of the child's behavior than the other. In short, you feel embarrassed, angry, and frustrated, and the cumulative toll on you and your whole family is immense.

Disruptive disorders are also often socially isolating for the child and the whole family as well. Parents who continually meet with resistance from their child are apt to find themselves in a self-perpetuating, tempestuous circle: The child fails to get ready for school or to comply with some other seemingly simple demand of daily life, and the parent becomes angry and frustrated, creating an environment that makes the child even less capable of focusing and getting ready. The bad behavior escalates, starting the next round of the cycle. In my office, I frequently deal with families who find themselves trying to cope with an impossible child who has no friends and is doing horribly in school—a child whom everyone hates, including them.

Despite all of the issues that surround disruptive disorders, it seems odd to think that they can be difficult to properly identify—after all, the behaviors that characterize them are hard to miss. However, the controversy that surrounds these diagnoses has to do with the degree to which the observed behaviors are voluntary, purposeful, or perhaps simply a matter of insufficient parental guidance or child motivation. Be honest: If you see a parent watching helplessly as a six- or seven-year-old boy runs amok in a store, loudly demanding that the parent buy him this or that, your first thought is probably not, "Ah, there's a boy with ADHD." Most of us tend to attribute such behaviors to bad parenting and, as I mentioned earlier, that often holds true for the parents themselves.

The fact that there is no definitive test for ADHD or other disruptive disorders further complicates the situation. The behaviors that we use to define these disorders are by no means specific to the disorder— they can arise from a variety of conditions or even represent normative behavior, depending on how often they occur, how severe they are, and why they happen. In these days of managed care, pediatricians often have limited opportunities for referral, and they are certainly limited in terms of time. A good number of them try to diagnose ADHD by putting a child on a stimulant such as methylphenidate (Ritalin) in the thoroughly disproven (but still popular) belief that if it works to slow the child down, then the child has ADHD. As you may have guessed, this is not the path to getting a proper diagnosis.

These disorders tend to coexist with other disorders, further complicating the situation. For example, oppositional defiant disorder (ODD) occurs in about 40 percent of kids with ADHD, with conduct disorder occurring in another 10 to 20 percent. Anxiety and depression also commonly occur in kids with ADHD, as do learning disorders. Furthermore, children with ADHD are far more likely than those without ADHD to experience trauma severe enough to cause chronic problems; it is not hard to imagine that their behaviors sometimes leads to physical abuse, adding another layer of problems.

The bulk of this chapter is devoted to issues concerning ADHD; not only is it the most common of the disruptive disorders, it is also such a buzzword among parents and educators that there is a great deal to address on the topic. The chapter concludes with a discussion of both oppositional defiant disorder and conduct disorder.

Attention-Deficit/ Hyperactivity Disorder

ADHD is a neurobiological disorder that affects 5 to 9 percent of school-age children. ADHD is characterized by inappropriate levels of inattention, impulsivity, and hyperactivity. If properly identified and treated, symptom reduction can be quite successful, and people with ADHD can have highly successful lives. However, if ADHD is never properly diagnosed and addressed, its symptoms can be life-disrupting and cause difficulties in school and with relationships.

Phrases like "I'm so A-D-H-D," or "I'm having an A-D-H-D moment" have become part of our vernacular, and are used by perfectly normal adults and adolescents to explain forgetfulness, inability to focus, or to excuse channel surfing or flitting in and out of online conversations. While people today use the term flippantly, fifteen years ago, ADHD was a shameful diagnosis: How could college-educated, "smart" people have children with ADHD? This disorder carries with it lots baggage and misunderstandings.

When I do media interviews about ADHD, I'm nearly always asked, "Is ADHD over- or underdiagnosed?" My typical answer is "yes." I go on to explain that research clearly shows that many children receiving stimulant medication do not have ADHD, and that many children with ADHD who could benefit from effective treatment never receive the diagnosis. As previously discussed, these failures to provide accurate diagnoses usually come from an inadequate assessment or no assessment at all.

Some critics have suggested that ADHD is a "school-induced diagnosis," meaning that school can be an especially difficult setting for children with this disorder. There is certainly some truth to the observation that ADHD is more disruptive and intolerable in some settings than in others; undoubtedly, there are also some teachers who would like their classrooms better if the most energetic children in it were quieter. This is worrisome. As we all know, children mature at different rates. The child in first grade who blurts out answers, squirms in her seat, and doesn't even seem to notice a class-

LIVING WITH CHILDREN WITH ADHD

Willie is a four-year- old boy whose mother brought him in to see me after the following particularly harrowing occurrence. One day, Willie's mother was watching Willie play with some toys in the family's living room, but left him alone briefly so she could go to the bathroom. When she returned a few minutes later, he was no longer in the living room. She searched every room in the house—quickly, because she'd learned that his being unsupervised was always a risk—until she finally found him in the kitchen. He'd decided to "make lunch." The refrigerator door was standing wide open with various items scattered on the floor. He had somehow gotten several eggs from the top door shelf, then climbed some drawers to get onto the electric stovetop, where he'd positioned himself atop one of the burners. He was turning one on when his mother found him—just in time.

When asked about his early developmental history, his mother laughingly recounted that Willie actually had never learned to "walk." One day, at age thirteen months, he lurched to his feet for the first time and barreled across the room at a fast pace until he rammed into the door frame, knocking himself unconscious. Willie was impulsive, seemed to have no sense of self-preservation, and could not stay focused on any activity for more than a few seconds. Attempts to put him into preschool were a disaster: He wrecked toys, bit other children, and generally motored around the playground, ignoring adults who tried to slow him down. Despite all that, he was a pleasant, well-meaning child with a higher-than-average intelligence. Willie's father, Bill, no longer in the picture, reportedly had been "just like Willie" when he was young. Bill had done poorly in school, never graduated from high school, and had a "wild adolescence"—but never got into any real trouble. As an adult, he held menial jobs, but never for long because he got bored. He'd been on Ritalin as a child but stopped taking it in early adolescence, a customary practice at the time.

Willie's story serves as a reminder that ADHD is not something that can be dealt with casually; and, if Willie's experience is similar to his father's, it's also not something he will outgrow—he'll be dealing with ADHD for the rest of his life.

mate in the doorway as she steamrolls out for recess may have ADHD or may simply be a little slower to mature than her classmates. Yet I also worry about the child with ADHD who just cannot follow the rules, and begins as early as kindergarten to get the message that he is bad because he doesn't.

Children with ADHD are sometimes inconsistent in their behaviors. For example, they'll sit happily watching their favorite action-adventure video but are "bouncing off the walls" in math class. This inconsistency leads adults to think the child is lazy or just badly behaved. (One book about ADHD is aptly titled, *You Mean I'm Not Lazy, Stupid or Crazy?!*) Children with ADHD experience delays in independent functioning. This poses a special challenge to teenagers, since they are already impulsive and have difficulty dealing with the typical adolescent issues of peer pressure, sexuality, avoiding drug abuse, etc. We expect more and more independence and self-reliance from them, and increasingly hold them to adult standards of behavior. For a teenager with ADHD, the added burdens of poor sustained attention with easy distractibility (often manifested as boredom) and impulsivity (often manifested as

THE OTHER ADHD

Suzanne was a quiet, dreamy child who never caused any trouble. Her parents brought her in to see me when she was eleven because her grades were rapidly slipping. She had done well enough in grade school, although her parents admitted that they always had to help her more than they thought they should, ensuring that she had the right books at home to do her projects, making certain she got her homework done, and even checking that she turned it in. When she started middle school, Suzanne's teachers told them she needed to be more responsible, so they stopped supervising her so closely. The result was an unhappy child, irritated teachers, and increasingly despondent parents. When they looked at the criteria for ADHD, she met all the ones for inattention and none for hyperactivity or impulsivity. Testing showed that she was of average intelligence and had no learning problems.

Helping Suzanne and her parents understand that she was not just lazy was an essential first step, as was reassessing what she needed to succeed in school. A small dose of a stimulant medication was all that was needed to help her focus considerably better in school, but she did not require medication on the weekends or holidays. Even with medication, parents and teachers still had to provide structure for her during the day and between school and home, but, with those adjustments, Suzanne became successful again.

poor judgment) can result in recurrent actions that fail to meet those standards.

What Is It?

ADHD is an inherited, potentially lifelong disorder that is characterized by persistent problems with attention, impulsivity, and overall activity levels. The most striking problems in younger individuals typically involve impulsive actions and constant movement. This is the preschooler who never sits still, is always exploring, probing, jumping, climbing. He's the one who hits or bites the child who asks to play with his toy, or the one who impulsively decides to climb the bookshelves and jump off "because it looked like fun." In older children with ADHD, hyperactivity and impulsivity may continue, but issues of attention and distractibility also become apparent. These are the children who never listen to instructions, who start a task but then leave it for something new that came up, who finish their homework—usually with lots of help from parents—but then fail to turn it in because it is wadded up and forgotten in the bottom of their overstuffed backpack.

During adolescence, hyperactivity may evolve into restlessness and boredom, but the impulsivity and distractibility can become even more apparent and problematic. At this point, experts become concerned about issues with executive function, which is the ability to form a plan to accomplish a series of tasks efficiently. Consider, for example, cooking an elaborate meal. You need to make sure in advance that all the ingredients you need are available and ensure you know in detail how each item is best prepared. You also have to schedule your preparation so each item is ready to eat at the appropriate time—and take the same care for several other recipes. People with ADHD may find such feats of planning difficult to impossible.

Individuals with ADHD also tend to have weak short-term memory, have difficulty making transitions, and show a limited ability to inhibit thoughts, speech, and actions (hence impulsivity). They may talk excessively, have trouble concentrating on repetitive tasks, and are easily diverted away from tasks requiring sustained concentration, such as homework. Some ADHD individuals have an amazing ability to "hyperfocus" on things that interest them—video games are a prime example. These games provide nonstop stimulation and have clear rewards for successful behavior; parents come into my office expressing disbelief at what the teacher may tell them about their child, "Because, Dr. Elliott, we know he can pay attention—the teacher just isn't engaging him."

Types of ADHD

Currently, ADHD is divided into three subtypes:

- **Mainly hyperactive/impulsive.** Children in this category are primarily fidgety, restless, and impetuous. This subtype is most commonly diagnosed in preschool children, probably because it is very difficult to assess attention at that age.
- **Mainly inattentive.** These children daydream, forget, and procrastinate, but they can sit still and aren't especially impulsive. This subtype is typically diagnosed later, often around the age of ten or twelve years, mainly because these problems don't worry other people until the children become older and need to be more self-sufficient.
- **Combined.** Some children exhibit symptoms from both subtypes; they are distractible, impulsive, and hyperactive.

This subtype is the most commonly diagnosed and most closely matches what used to be called "hyperactivity."

Until recently, few teachers, pediatricians, and mental health professionals working with children and adolescents knew how to recognize symptoms of the inattentive subtype of ADHD. Although boys still outnumber girls, the male-to-female ratio is much closer to equal than for the other two subtypes, where boys are three to four times more numerous. Girls generally seem to manifest less disruptive symptoms and are therefore less likely to catch negative attention from the teacher. They are the ones the teacher may be disappointed in because they are sitting quietly in the back of the room, not causing trouble but also not participating—and quite possibly not absorbing enough information.

There is still a lot to learn about inattentive ADHD. Currently, most of what we know about the inattentive and distractible subtype comes from studies of combined-type ADHD. Studying children who only have inattentive symptoms will increase our knowledge considerably; perhaps the problems these children have processing information is related to the trouble they have staying on task. Hopefully, studies of treatment interventions for this subtype of ADHD, which lags far behind those for combined-type ADHD, will also increase.

What the Statistics Tell Us

Children between the ages of six and eight are the most studied group with ADHD. Research has shown that combined-type ADHD is often diagnosed between these ages; the inattentive type is usually found in children aged eight to eleven. ADHD becomes increasingly obvious and impairing by middle school, when expectations for independence increase and when other children are acquiring skills. In the short run, these children respond well to medications and behavioral interventions, but these options do not change the underlying problem. The disorder is still present, but children have fewer symptoms while on medication—just as aspirin doesn't cure a fever but makes you feel better. In addition, researchers have yet to show that any interventions currently available reliably change the course of the illness, however well they may do in the short term.

Doctors used to think that children outgrew ADHD, since hyperactivity typically lessens during the teen years. We now know that ADHD symptoms are present in one- to two-thirds of adolescents and adults who had ADHD as children. That means that roughly 2 to 4 percent of adults continue to have marked problems because of ADHD, and their impairments can be serious. Problems with academic achievement, driving, drug and alcohol use, unsafe sex, relationships with peers, work, and legal issues are common in adults with ADHD. Teenagers with ADHD are also at a higher risk for substance abuse. These youth are twice as likely to become addicted to nicotine as individuals without ADHD, and as adults, they have elevated smoking rates and difficulty quitting. Adolescents who are taking stimulants appear to be less likely to use illegal drugs than those who are not taking medications, but this data remains controversial.

Seldom the Only Issue

ADHD rarely appears in isolation, and a comprehensive evaluation is necessary to rule out other causes and to determine the presence or absence of coexisting conditions. Other disruptive behaviors often accompany ADHD: About 40 percent of individuals with ADHD have

ODD. Conduct disorder is also more likely to be found in children with ADHD.

Another common companion to ADHD is depression; 10 to 30 percent of children with ADHD are also depressed. Whether this is genetic or environmental is unclear—certainly the ADHD child often finds himself left out on the playground, dropped off birthday party guest lists, and not invited on playdates and sleepovers. This may occur because he's a "handful," and the schoolmates' parents don't want to deal with it, or sometimes because the hyperactive or impulsive qualities are socially disruptive. A child constantly interrupting in the midst of a game, suddenly trying to lift up a playmate, or not being able to focus on a particular activity can create a situation where his or her peers simply don't like having the child around. As these negative social episodes pile up, the child is left feeling isolated and sad, and that can certainly contribute to depression.

As many as 30 percent of children with ADHD also have an anxiety disorder. These kids often don't exhibit hyperactivity, but they do have trouble functioning and have more problems with school and social interactions. In general, they are described as "slowed down" and inefficient. For these children, paying attention to stressors and working on relaxation techniques can be helpful. Those who are anxious may have more variable responses to stimulants such as methylphenidate, and alternative medications should be considered.

ADHD and a tendency for tics (sudden rapid recurrent nonrhythmic movements or vocalizations) or Tourette's syndrome (physical tics and analogous vocal tics) are clearly linked, although the mechanism is not understood. Only about 7 percent of those with ADHD have tics or Tourette's syndrome, but 60 percent of those with Tourette's have ADHD.

One very controversial topic related to ADHD is the possible overlap with bipolar disorder. Bipolar disorder is a psychiatric condition that, in adults, results in episodes of either extremely elevated or depressed moods, along with other changes in appetite, thinking, sleep, etc. Some clinical researchers have argued that, although bipolar disorder typically does not become apparent until adulthood, it may influence behavior at much younger ages. They also suggest that it may look just like ADHD: Impulsive behavior, high physical activity, poor attention, and a cranky or irritable mood are common to both disorders.

According to researchers, nearly one in four children now diagnosed as having ADHD actually has bipolar disorder. Those who are diagnosed with ADHD but actually have bipolar disorder are not only apt to respond poorly to conventional ADHD medications, but actually may do much worse because of such treatments. It is believed that these children respond well to medications that are helpful in treating adult bipolar disorder, but there is a frustrating lack of evidence for this. I believe it is a far less common problem than the advocates suggest, and most families are better served seeking help for ADHD first. If responses are atypical or inadequate, then it is wise to look for alternative explanations.

ADHD and Learning Disabilities

About a third of children with ADHD also have a coexisting learning disorder, usually a specific problem with reading or calculating. This does not mean that they are less intelligent than their peers; they just have specific weaknesses in learning. Students with both ADHD and dyslexia, a reading disorder, are no more anxious, hyperactive, or aggressive than students with ADHD only. Learning disabilities can affect school performance, however, and the combination can make life more difficult for the child. The inability to stay focused makes overcoming the learning problem more difficult, and the extra effort needed to overcome the learning problem makes it tempting to give in to impulsive urges.

If you are concerned that your child may have a learning problem, contact the school principal, teacher, or guidance department. Schools are mandated by law to formally explore these concerns and assess all children for learning disabilities. Medications do not treat these issues specifically, but they may improve other symptoms so that learning can accelerate.

To deal more successfully with coexisting conditions, families must:
- Consider that some children will improve with effective treatment of ADHD
- Recognize that other issues, such as learning disabilities and language disorders, may not improve in the same way
- Create a hierarchy of response to all symptoms, using best judgment about which issues are primary (for example, is anxiety or depression a result of ADHD, or simply creating overlapping symptoms?)

What Causes It?

According to most researchers, ADHD is a complex brain-based disorder. Its exact cause is still unknown, but genetic and neurobiological vulnerabilities are being explored as potential options. It almost certainly is not a single-cause disorder; it develops from a variety of factors. There is strong evidence that the disorder is genetic, and environment may contribute to its manifestation in those who are sensitive to environmental influences. Fetal alcohol syndrome (negative effects on the unborn child due to alcohol consumed during pregnancy), other drug effects in utero, and lead levels in the blood during early childhood have all been linked to ADHD.

The search for the underlying brain mechanisms that cause ADHD is ongoing. The best available evidence implicates a chemical messenger in the brain called dopamine, which tells our brain what in the environment is important and valuable, and what we can afford to ignore. Research suggests that people with ADHD don't have enough dopamine in the part of the brain that controls cognitive skills, such as forming a plan or controlling reactions to outside events.

A factor with almost every psychiatric disorder or behavioral problem is the issue of nature versus nurture, and ADHD is no exception. Does a chaotic, disorganized household create children with ADHD, or does ADHD induce chaos in the household? The answer is unclear, and it may well be caused by a bit of both. While a chaotic home environment may not be the primary cause, we do know that a calm and controlled atmosphere helps provide the type of structure helpful for those with ADHD. In addition, given the disorder's genetic component, it is not unusual to find a household where more than one member has ADHD, which may itself add to the chaos.

The great increase in the use of methylphenidate to treat ADHD, especially in the U.S., has led to a concern that parents are using the ADHD diagnosis as a way to medicate children who are only somewhat difficult or simply active, because they don't have the patience to deal with them. Consider an alternate view: Compared to previous generations, children enter out-of-home situations (like preschools) earlier and more often than before. These settings may bring to light ADHD-related problems that may not have been otherwise detected, and allow children to get the help they need. Still, it is more likely that preschool teachers will accommodate children who are always moving and unable to stay on a task for long than are teachers in elementary schools.

The Diagnosis

Most families begin the ADHD evaluation process by asking their pediatrician about their child's excessive activity or inability to focus on one thing. If the child isn't in school yet, the doctor will most likely reassure parents that it's too early to tell. In most cases, it makes sense to wait a while and see if a child calms down as she matures. However, if she's about to get kicked out of preschool or already failing kindergarten, then simply hoping she'll resist the urge to bite a child the next time she's frustrated won't help much. If there is reason for concern, you are better off getting a referral to someone who specializes in these evaluations.

This evaluation should include both a careful history and clinical assessment of academic, social, and emotional functioning, as well as developmental level. Both parents and teachers should fill out a detailed questionnaire to help form a more complete picture of the child's situation. The pediatrician should conduct a complete physical in order to rule out any health problems, including hearing or vision difficulties and thyroid dysfunction. Physical causes are rare, but missing them can be tragic.

In retrospect, parents may realize that their child showed early symptoms of ADHD but, particularly with a first child, they may be hard-pressed to know what normal is. Children who will one day be diagnosed as ADHD may be very demanding as babies—they cry during feedings and having trouble settling into a comfortable sucking rhythm. They may be colicky and dislike being held. As they graduate to real food, they may be picky eaters. These children often develop self-soothing behaviors such as thumb-sucking, head-banging, or rocking back and forth. Once mobile, they may be in constant motion, and parents may find themselves continually on alert, not knowing whether the child will decide to try to

WHAT'S TO BLAME?

Over the past fifty years, there have been many theories about the likely causes of ADHD, especially the possibility that it results from being "poisoned" by the presence or absence of certain substances in modern food. For example, highly processed foods were thought to lack essential elements or contain additives, such as dyes or preservatives, that made children hyper. Similarly, some parents observed that their child would get particularly out of control when exposed to refined sugars or artificial sweeteners. Most physicians, including myself, regard such theories with considerable skepticism. There are individual cases, however, especially with pre-school-age children, in which dietary changes are beneficial. It is difficult to judge whether the sometimes severe dietary restrictions needed to produce change are the best approach to helping the average child with ADHD. I tell families that this is not a treatment I usually advise, because I have not been impressed with the results. If they wish to pursue such options, they are welcome to do so elsewhere and come back to me if it doesn't work for their child.

scale a bookcase or make a break for the front door.

ADHD by the Book

The *Diagnostic and Statistical Manual of Mental Disorders, 4th Edition* presents the following list of possible symptoms for ADHD. Clinicians work with the child, parents, and teachers to determine how many symptoms a child has. To consider ADHD as a possible diagnosis, they must identify six symptoms from either or both of the subtypes; each must be consistently present for a period of at least six months, and there must be no better explanation for why they occur. Since ADHD is thought to exist from birth, another requirement is that symptoms must be present by at least age seven, even if the diagnosis is made later.

Criteria for the hyperactive/impulsive subtype include:

- Fidgeting or squirming
- Difficulty remaining seated
- Running or climbing excessively
- Difficulty engaging in activities quietly
- Acting as if driven by a motor
- Talking excessively
- Blurting out answers before questions have been completed
- Difficulty waiting or taking turns
- Interrupting or intruding upon others

Criteria for the inattentive/distractible subtype include:

- Failing to pay close attention to details or making careless mistakes
- Difficulty sustaining attention
- Appearing not to listen

- Struggling to follow through on instructions
- Difficulty with organization
- Avoiding or disliking tasks requiring sustained mental effort
- Losing things
- Being easily distracted
- Being forgetful in daily activities

Children with the combined subtype meet at least six of the nine criteria for both of the other subtypes.

Normal Toddler or ADHD?

Because "active," "on the go," and "impulsive" are the very definitions of being a toddler, diagnosing ADHD in preschool children is difficult. What makes the ADHD child different is that he continues to run instead of walk, switches from one thing to another impulsively, has a temper tantrum when taken away from something he does find interesting, and refuses to sit through a story long after his peers are learning what proper behavior is. It is not clear whether these children are incapable of perceiving social clues or just ignoring them.

When these children enter elementary school, excessively agitated behavior becomes more visible and more unacceptable, as compared to other children. Teachers will notice that conduct is bad and schoolwork shows problems. The child may appear not to listen and will likely have difficulty organizing thoughts or participating in anything that requires sustained attention. Many have difficulty with sequential memory (remembering things in order) and sometimes have trouble with fine motor skills. Unfortunately, many of these kids end up in trouble more often than not and this, combined with the difficulty with schoolwork, means that their self-esteem suffers.

Treatment

While some families prefer to exhaust other options before putting a child on medication, more than two hundred studies have shown that medication can produce striking results for those diagnosed with ADHD. Use of medications for treating ADHD has skyrocketed, jumping about 23 percent between 2000 and 2003, according to a study of 300,000 members of pharmacy-benefit manager Medco Health Solutions, Inc. Young patients with this disorder generally respond well to both stimulants and several nonstimulant medications. Statistically, 65 to 85 percent of children with ADHD have a positive response, and experience an increase in attention and concentration, decreased physical activity and impulsivity, enhanced compliance and effort on tasks, and improved accuracy. They also experience a decrease in negative behaviors and physical and verbal hostility.

In addition to improving classroom behavior and academic focus, medications can also have a positive social value. Through a combination of medication and behavior therapy, children start to experience fewer impulsive behaviors, are better liked by their peers, are punished less frequently in the classroom, and can start to establish a better self-image.

Stimulants

By far the best-studied area in all of child and adolescent psychopharmacology is the use of stimulants, the most common class of medication prescribed for ADHD, on children between the ages of seven and eleven years. Stimulant-type medications have been in use since the late 1930s, but became prominent in the 1960s with the introduction of methylphenidate, more commonly known as Ritalin. Today, stimulant medications consist primarily of some form of methylphenidate or amphetamine, and there are several variations of each that differ in how they are prepared. These differences affect how long the drug acts during the day and the pattern of its release.

While the idea of giving a stimulant to someone who is already hyper seems counterintuitive, the fact is that these medications increase attention and reduce

excess fidgeting and hyperactivity. They are thought to work by increasing the activity of the neurotransmitters (chemical messengers in the brain) dopamine and norepinephrine, which in turn increases nervous system alertness. The effect usually occurs within a half hour after the first dose and can be quite dramatic. Children are quieter and less impulsive, able to concentrate longer, less influenced by distractions, better able to complete tasks, and more likely to listen to and comply with requests. The effect lasts as long as the medication is in the system and it diminishes as the medicine leaves the body. The most common side effects of stimulants are reduced appetite, difficulty falling asleep, and occasionally headaches and stomachaches, particularly in the beginning. These can generally be corrected by reducing the dosage.

Choosing to put a child on stimulants is a serious decision and you should consider the following factors:
- Severity of the disorder
- Availability of feasible alternatives
- Short- and long-term benefits of the medication
- Possible side effects

As mentioned earlier, some pediatricians put children on a stimulant medication as a test to see if the child has

ADHD. As easy an answer as this may seem, it is wrong for several reasons. First, all prepubescent children react somewhat similarly to stimulants—they become more attentive, less distractible, less impulsive, and physically less active. These reactions do not amount to a diagnosis of ADHD. Between 15 and 35 percent of children with ADHD will not respond well to any stimulant, so a poor response cannot serve as proof the child does not have ADHD. Most importantly, however, is the fact that every child deserves a thorough diagnosis, and not one based on guesswork.

Age plays a large role in children's reactions to stimulants. Even though there has been a huge increase in the amount of stimulants being prescribed for children under six, very little is known about their safety and efficacy for this age group. The first-ever long-term study was completed in 2005, and information from this study indicates that stimulants do not generally have notably worse or different side effects than in older children, but seem to be less effective overall.

Once a child enters adolescence, it is important to reassess whether ADHD symptoms persist and what approaches will be the most effective. Again, we know far less about the use of stimulants for ADHD in this age group than for younger children. There are two issues particularly relevant for adolescents, and the first has to do with noncompliance. Teenagers need to assert their independence, and often this results in a refusal to take medication regularly or at all. This idea usually occurs just at the point when the academic load is getting heavier, and so the child who has been maintaining As and Bs may suddenly be unable to focus in class or on tests, and grades take a precipitous drop. Alert parents and teachers may be able to counteract this rebellion, but it isn't always easy. The second concern is drug abuse. Available evidence suggests that well-diagnosed adolescents are relatively unlikely to abuse stimulants—as one teenager put it, "What's the fun of taking a drug that calms you down?" However, they have an increased risk of using and abusing other drugs. They may also become targets of peers who want the adolescent to give them his or her stimulant medications so they can abuse them.

Behavior Management

As useful as medication can be for many children, it almost never is the sole solution to the problems ADHD can cause. Behavior management can also be a large part of the process. Frequently, families get to a place where the child feels like a "bad kid," and parents are constantly frustrated. Behavior management can help wipe the family slate clean and get everyone off to a better start. Educating parents about the key features of ADHD throughout life and how that affects their child's parenting needs can be of considerable value.

The Multimodal Treatment of ADHD (MTA) Study

In 1989, the National Institute of Mental Health (NIMH) began funding a landmark study called the Multimodal Treatment Study of Children with ADHD (MTA). I have been involved in this study from its inception, and it has continually provided enormous amounts of information about ADHD as it follows children from latency (ages six to eight) to young adulthood. The study involved 579 children with combined-type ADHD. Each child re-

---

ALTERNATE ROUTES

Because of recent concerns about side effects and the long-term use of medications, people have been looking for other solutions. The number of alternative methods is burgeoning, but while companies may proclaim anecdotal success, these methods typically have little to no research to back up their claims. They also tend to be very expensive. Here are some of the methods being used:

- The **Tomatis Method**, begun in France in the 1950s, uses music to help children learn to focus, and the company reports that it can improve attention and listening skills. It gained a following in the U.S. in the early 1990s and there are now several centers throughout the country.

- The **Brain Gym** teaches exercise and movement that is designed to develop and coordinate the brain. The program is an outgrowth of Educational Kinesiology Foundation in Ventura, California, and their mission is to train teachers around the country.

- **Dore Achievement Centers** offer an intervention that uses brain-stimulating exercises to try to improve brain functioning and increase the attention span.

- **EEG training** asserts that teaching children with ADHD to alter their brain waves with bio-feedback helps control ADHD symptoms. The ability to deliberately change EEG waves in a controlled setting is well documented, but it is unclear if it can affect day-to-day symptoms.

- **Herbal supplements** (such as Pynogemin, a high-potency vitamin C supplement with added vitamins or Focus ADHD Formula) and **homeopathic medicine** (such as Attend) are also being used as natural remedies for ADHD. These have not undergone rigorous clinical trials, since the U.S. Congress does not require the FDA to monitor food supplements.

ceived one of four possible treatments over a fourteen-month period—medication management, behavioral treatment, a combination of the two, or usual community care ranging from no care at all to medications prescribed by a pediatrician.

The results of the study showed that the best outcomes at the end of fourteen months of treatment came from the groups of children who were treated with medication alone (carefully managed and individually tailored), and the children who received both carefully managed medication and behavioral guidance. Overall, the combined treatment provided the best results, with the major initial effect resulting from medication. Surprisingly, Ritalin not only helped with ADHD symptoms, it also decreased problems related to ODD, anxiety, and depression. The children in combined treatment did especially well in their interactions with their parents. The study revealed that both the dosage and timing of the medication must be carefully calculated in order to have the maximum benefit. The study also showed that for those opposed to medication, behavior management can be effective. However, it requires very focused and consistent effort on the part of the parents and teachers.

The behavioral interventions that work are consistent, targeted, meaningfully positive, timely, and reinforced ones. This kind of intervention should be accompanied by cognitive behavioral therapy, social skills training, parent education and support, and remedial education. Success in school may also require a variety of classroom accommodations. Two federal laws—the Individuals with Disabilities Education Act (IDEA) and Section 504 of the Rehabilitation Act of 1973—guarantee children with ADHD a free and appropriate public education.

Oppositional Defiant Disorder

As hard as children with ADHD can be to parent, the problems they cause can pale when compared with the parenting challenges that children and adolescents with oppositional defiant disorder or conduct disorder (CD) pose. These children seem to thrive on conflict and rule violations, and parents grow both exhausted and humiliated at their failure to get them to understand the rules, let alone obey them. Although learning that you are not alone in this struggle can be an enormous relief, that knowledge is only the beginning of the battle. These disorders, more than any others in child psychiatry, require a commitment from the parents to change how they interact with their child. The work focuses as much on giving parents support and new parenting skills as on changing the child's behaviors.

What Is It?

Most children are oppositional (openly uncooperative and hostile) at times, but if a pattern of such disruptive behavior develops and persists, then a child may be diagnosed with ODD. Most commonly, children with ODD are "strong-willed" or irritable, and they do not like being told what to do, usually from an early age. ODD often appears to result from a combination of child temperament and parenting style. Both experience and research suggest that some children would be oppositional regardless of parenting style; others are so mellow that even the worst problems rarely make them oppositional. For most children, however, the problem is neither a bad temperament nor terrible parents—just a bad mix.

Symptoms of ODD may include:

- Frequent temper tantrums
- Excessive arguing with adults
- Active defiance and refusal to comply with adult requests and rules
- Deliberate attempts to annoy or upset people
- Blaming others for his or her mistakes or misbehavior
- Being touchy or easily annoyed by others
- Frequent anger and resentment
- Mean and hateful response when upset
- Seeking revenge

In order to be diagnosed with this disorder, these behaviors must occur in multiple settings and not simply be the result of a conflict with a particular parent or teacher. In some cases, older children with ODD start out as fussy, colicky, difficult infants and may have pushed the limits during the "terrible twos," had frequent temper tantrums, and caused difficulty around issues such as eating, toilet training, sleeping, and speaking. Many are taken in for hearing evaluations as they seem not to hear; however, the issue usually involves not listening.

Some might worry that during the teenage years many of the ODD symptoms can be mistaken for normal adolescence, and it certainly is important to consider these behaviors with the developmental process in mind. Still, many with ODD develop in a previously established pattern— they break rules because they are there or force negative and defeatist interactions with authority figures. They seem to say, "I win because you lose," or, "If I lose, it's never my fault."

Children with mild ODD may only erupt at home, while at school they passively resist cooperating and aren't necessarily openly hostile. Instead, they will avoid saying "no" outright yet constantly dawdle and procrastinate—the intent is the same. ODD diagnosed before puberty is seen far more frequently in boys than in girls; after puberty, the diagnoses of boys and girls becomes about equal.

What Causes It?

As previously mentioned, ODD seems to result from a bad fit between a child's needs and the caretaker's parenting style. A fussy or colicky baby may put parents' nerves on edge, then parental tension begins to enter into the family dynamics, and the baby or toddler becomes fearful and difficult to deal with. When parents start to assert control in areas like eating, toilet training, sleeping, or speaking politely, the child resists. The parents' sense of inefficacy increases, as does overall family negativism. Soon, the parents respond to the child in anger, and a pattern is established. The problems increase, and the pattern may start to spread outside the home.

In school, these children are often disruptive—banging books on desks, refusing to line up for gym class, or claiming they aren't going to do the homework. With chronic criticism directed at them, they begin to feel badly about themselves, which lowers their self-esteem; conversely, they may see themselves as successful in the interminable wars they ignite. Many feel victimized and unfairly picked on. Frequently, these children have other issues ranging from OCD or ADHD to depression or even mania.

Of course, biological and genetic factors may also play a role in ODD. For example, children with ADHD have a far greater likelihood of also having ODD than those without ADHD. Still, biological factors seem to relate to a child's vulnerability for developing ODD, rather than being a direct cause of the disorder.

The Diagnosis

It is important to emphasize that an ODD diagnosis is not appropriate for children who occasionally get into bad moods or are set off by a particular authority figure. Who hasn't had that experience? ODD reflects a consistent pattern in which the relationships a child has with others, especially adults, is characterized by negativity and resistance. When asked to sit, he wants to stand; when told to stop playing in five minutes, he insists on an hour. No issue is too small to engender an argument, and no limit is too minor to breach.

Treatment

There is no medication for ODD, but a professional evaluation can still be quite helpful. The child may also be suffering from other concurrent disorders, such as ADHD or depression, that medication may be beneficial for. The family will need to work on creating a new and more positive environment. Change is possible, but the whole family must participate. Parents need to regain the control they've lost over the child and the situation, while the child needs to learn that parents can effectively provide positive responses for desirable behaviors. The child needs consistent, clear, and meaningful rules and expectations to help clarify the parent-child relationship. A professional will be able to help parents and children relate better, and individual psychotherapy, family therapy, parent- training programs, and the coordination of a reward program may all prove helpful.

Conduct Disorder

Individuals, mainly adolescents, who have conduct disorder are prone to committing serious rule violations that may involve any of the following:

- **Aggression toward people and animals** (bullying, intimidation, initiating physical fights, physical cruelty, assault, or sexual assault)
- **Destruction of property** (starting fires, deliberate destruction)
- **Deceitfulness** (lying, stealing, shoplifting, staying out all night, running away, truancy, breaking and entering)

What Is It?

Conduct disorder is what used to be called delinquency. These are children who break the rules because they can—they don't think the rules really apply to them. About 6 percent of all children have some form of conduct disorder, and it usually emerges during adolescence. Many suffered from ODD when they were younger, but discovered during adolescence that beyond conflict with other individuals are numerous societal rules that are just waiting to be broken. As a result, these children may end up in either the mental health system or the legal system—sometimes both. In younger populations, CD occurs almost exclusively in boys, but more and more girls join the group as adolescence progresses. CD is commonly found in poor inner-city areas, along with high rates of family instability, social disorganization, infant morbidity and mortality, and severe illness.

Conduct disorder is complicated. The child who has difficulty following rules is generally viewed as bad or delinquent rather than mentally ill. It is upsetting to all family members, and difficult for parents because of the child's apparent lack of remorse or even an understanding of the damage inflicted on others.

Some studies suggest that there are two broad groups of people with CD, although they can be hard to identify at a quick glance. One type stems from having ODD as a child which progresses into CD in early adolescence, with increased reckless and defiance of social constraints. Many such individuals continue this behavior into adulthood, often with lives full of destructive behaviors. The other group appears normal as children (even in retrospect), but go wild during adolescence—breaking rules, taking chances, and "sowing their wild oats." Research suggests that many in this latter group grow out of these behaviors sometime in their early twenties—if they have not destroyed themselves before then. Those who avoid potentially permanent dead ends have a real chance of living a normal, productive life.

Children with CD misbehave to express distress caused by anger, frustration, disappointment, anxiety, or sorrow. As they grow up, it is assumed that their behavior will improve and they won't need to act out anymore, but this is a potentially damaging assumption. If the unacceptable behavior goes on for too long, the child may end up committing an act that is at best isolating, or at worst illegal or injurious. These children have a higher likelihood of turning to alcohol and drugs to "self-medicate" for anxiety, depression, thought disorders, hyperactivity, or insomnia, or to blot out memories of abuse. They often become cold and detached, lack empathy, and exhibit both suicidal behavior and aggression toward others. Without help, these children may not be able to become functioning adults.

The earlier a child displays extremely disturbed behavior, the easier it is to provide effective help. If the child is unmanageable by age four, then the situation is only going to get worse. If you are the parent of such a child and haven't yet sought help, do so.

What Causes It?

Researchers believe that children who develop conduct disorder have a biochemical and genetic vulnerability that makes them more susceptible when certain environmental issues come into play. These environmental triggers can include brain damage, child abuse, school failure, extreme poverty, or a traumatic experience. Sometimes the ability to identify and express emotions or an ineffective use of language may contribute to an inability to articulate feelings. This can lead a frustrated child to resort to physical expression to communicate. Unidentified learning disabilities may play a role in susceptibility to CD, and ADHD, depression, or bipolar disorder may also be concurrent.

The Diagnosis

When conduct disorder occurs before a child turns ten, it is referred to as childhood-onset conduct disorder. Adolescent-onset conduct disorder is more common. If you suspect your child has CD, then he or she will need a full evaluation, including a medical history, a family profile, and psychological testing. A clinician will look for repetitive and persistent patterns of rule violation, as well as a lack of empathy or understanding of wrongdoing. The neurological portion of the exam may include an EEG or MRI to test for central nervous system dysfunction, and a psychoeducational evaluation may uncover intellectual or learning disabilities that may put a child at additional risk for truancy and disruptive behaviors.

Treatment

Treatment for conduct disorder is complex and challenging, primarily because the patient is often uncooperative. While there is an increasing tendency to view these children as untreatable, this ignores the fact that many of them have serious underlying emotional disorders. Behavior therapy, psychotherapy, and, occasionally, medication may be used. Regardless of the therapy involved, long-term treatment will be necessary.

Since conduct issues tend to arise from a tangle of biological, emotional, and social stressors, no one class of medications is especially helpful. Lithium, a mood stabilizer, and anticonvulsant medications such as carbamazepine (Tegretol) have been shown to reduce aggression, at least in some individuals. If another psychiatric disorder (for example, ADHD, bipolar disorder, depression, or anxiety) is diagnosed, treating that disorder with medication may be helpful, but is unlikely to correct everything. Medication can also enhance the effectiveness of other treatments, such as parent management training, family therapy, social skills training, school-based treatment, and cognitive behavioral therapy.

Some have argued that conduct disorder is truly a product of our times, and that certain individuals simply cannot handle the complexities of modern life. Proponents of this theory recommend treatment programs that include a simplified lifestyle, spending time on an old-fashioned working farm or ranch in a rural setting, where the individual can learn to function in society better. A number of these centers have shown substantial benefits for the adolescents while they are in the program. However, it is more difficult to provide them with skills they can use in the "real world."

In the past decade, society has again

grown tired of coddling these children, and most states now have juvenile-offender facilities filled to capacity. As satisfying as such a punitive response may be to society's sense of self-righteousness, the evidence strongly suggests that this is an expensive approach which only winds up supporting habitual offenders jailed at the state's expense for the rest of their lives—when they are not out committing crimes.

The Bottom Line

Disruptive disorders can be stigmatizing for patient and parent alike. Considerable progress has been made in understanding and recognizing ADHD, and an array of treatment options promise some measure of success. However, controversies about the legitimacy of ADHD and effective treatment continue to abound. There is even less consensus about ODD and CD—why children have these disorders, and what to do about them.

If your child has a disruptive disorder, persevere and never give up. These are chronic, persistent disorders that require consistent, sustained interventions. Short-term gains often are surprisingly easy; harder by far are long-term solutions. You need to find someone you can trust and who will work with you not only for a few weeks, but for years.

Chapter 5

Affective Disorders

We have a tendency, both as individuals and as a society, to characterize childhood and adolescence as a happy time. This rose-colored view is probably a combination of selective memories from our own early years and wishing the best, if with a touch of envy, for the current generation. Whatever the reason, many adults find it hard to believe that children might actually suffer from sustained sadness. We all know that children have fleeting disappointments and occasional frustrations—but true depression?

It is easy for adults to overlook or dismiss the symptoms of childhood depression. Children don't always exhibit the symptoms of depression the same way adults do, and they are much more likely than adults to look depressed at some times and fine at others. In addition, especially with adolescents, it can be easy to write off disturbing behaviors as part of normal development rather than as signs of a worrisome disorder.

The medical and mental health professions have also been slow to recognize depression in the young. Only thirty years ago, psychiatry textbooks taught that depression did not occur before the mid- to late teen years. Researchers and clinicians willing to look at old phenomena in new ways discovered what now seems obvious: Depression can be serious, debilitating, even life-threatening, at all ages.

"What does my child have to be depressed about?" is a common question parents ask me. These parents are usually already well aware of the signs of depression: restlessness, agitation, persistent irritability, hypersensitivity, decreased concentration, changes in appetite and sleep, and a loss of enthusiasm about life. Such behaviors are why they find themselves in my office. And yet they find the possibility that their child is depressed baffling and unsettling.

When does sadness or disappointment become depression? Everyone gets upset, distressed, or sad sometimes, and we all respond to life events in very different ways. For some children, divorce, the death of a grandparent, a good friend moving away, or parental job loss may be issues that cause temporary sadness and regret—

and then they move on. For others, a single incident may be enough to trigger a disturbing or long-lasting mood disorder. And like adults, children sometimes become depressed for no obvious external reason. The distinguishing characteristics between "the blues" and an actual affective or mood disorder are duration, intensity, and pervasiveness. If sadness or symptoms that arise out of sadness last for more than a couple of weeks and interfere with normal functioning, then it is appropriate to consult your pediatrician.

In this chapter, I'll explain different types of affective, or mood, disorders. These include the two basic types of depression (major depression and the milder dysthymic disorder), and bipolar disorder (also known as manic-depressive illness). Adults with bipolar disorder have sustained periods of very "high" or manic time, and other sustained "low"

LIVING WITH A CHILD WITH A MOOD DISORDER

As the parent of a child with a serious affective disorder, you have almost certainly experienced an array of intense emotions yourself, including anger, frustration, self-doubt, helplessness, and fear. You may have watched your beautiful daughter lose interest in her friends, school, and life. You may have been baffled when your son, recently sobbing to you about how horrible he feels, suddenly brightens when friends show up unexpectedly. You may have found yourself going over all the items in the house that might be a weapon your child could use against himself. Is she using drugs? Is he safe to drive? Who can you tell? Will anyone—can anyone—help?

Parents with a depressed child may fantasize that mania must be better, but if you have a manic child or adolescent, you know that is not the case. Most young people with mania are irritable, not happy. They are full of energy and life, but you see how little it brings them. They never seem to sleep, and you worry about what they are doing in those waking hours. You watch as their friends pull away, frightened or offended. You see grades plummet, resources dwindle, and you fear that anything you say might set off another episode of rage. What should you do?

Even dysthymia (minor depression) is hard on parents. Your child never seems to find real joy in anything. If there is a negative perspective, she'll find it. It's like your son is wading through some sort of invisible, viscous fluid that slows him down but doesn't stop him. Is it just the way he is? Does she have a problem? Could it be that you've just forgotten what it's like to be a kid? Who can help you?

or depressed periods. In children, bipolar disorder is a bit more complicated. Because affective disorders tend to be recurrent and can be chronic, they can have a significant detrimental impact on all areas of children's lives; this makes accurate diagnosis and treatment critical. Because there is a similarity to treatment approaches for mood disorders, the chapter concludes with additional information on various forms of treatment.

Major Depression

What Is It?

A major depression is defined as a severe mood change, including symptoms of sadness or irritability that last for more than two weeks and have an impact on one's ability to function normally. Because "being depressed" is a term used casually for a wide range of emotional states, most people feel they know what it means to be depressed. A teen may get "depressed" for getting an A– instead of an A, or finding out it is too cold to go to the beach. Parents may say that their eight-year-old son is "depressed" because his best friend couldn't spend the night. Certainly, children of all ages can get "depressed" if a close friend moves away abruptly or if a pet dies. These are common reactions that may range in intensity and duration but typically last only minutes to days and seem appropriate to the occasion.

Mental health professionals use the term "depression" to refer to a syndrome that only partly has to do with mood. Beyond feelings of sadness or irritability, an individual may experience other characteristic changes in behavior that markedly interfere with daily life. These changes in mood and behavior are more severe, more impairing, and more sustained than would be considered reasonable for any individual.

Children exhibit the same range of signs and symptoms of depression that adults do. However, some of the more common symptoms differ, as children are much more likely than adults to be reactive to their environment. When they are busy with friends and engaged in activities they find interesting, they may seem fine, only to change abruptly as soon as their friends are out of sight. I once had a sixteen-year-old patient, Bryce, who had been profoundly depressed for two years and unresponsive to all treatment. His family used to live in Hawaii, and he had the chance to return there for a summer. Bryce reported that his depression lifted the instant he stepped off the airplane in Honolulu, and he had a wonderful time there, symptom free, for two months. To his—and my—amazement and dismay, his depression returned, full force, two weeks after he returned.

Identifying Depression

Identifying depression can be difficult, particularly with younger children. Researchers discovered that asking a seven- or eight-year-old child if she was depressed often led to a prompt "no," simply because that wasn't a term the child was familiar with. If the child felt "down," "sad," "blue," or "down in the dumps," it might simply not occur to her that that was the same thing as "depressed."

Depressed children may exhibit any of the following symptoms, which are a change from their normal behavior:

- Change in energy level, usually a decrease
- Decreased interest in activities—things that used to be fun no longer matter
- Frequent complaints about physical ailments such as headaches or stomachaches
- Difficulty concentrating
- Irritability which may manifest as bullying
- Significant increase or decrease in appetite leading to weight gain or loss
- Major changes in sleeping habits— either unable to sleep for long periods or suddenly sleeping for as many as fourteen hours

- Feelings of worthlessness
- Agitation
- Suicidal thoughts or attempts

Major depression usually interferes with social and academic functioning. Also, a decided change in a child's ability to keep up or stay involved with the things that are normally a part of his life can lead to a drop in self-esteem. More rarely, depression can become so severe that it produces psychosis. Children or adolescents might hear voices telling them how worthless they are or believe that parts of their bodies are decaying. They may even see things that aren't there, like rotting corpses.

Adolescents and Depression

Depression is sometimes overlooked in adolescents because our culture accepts teenage moodiness as a rite of passage. While it is true that the teenage years are a time of emotional upheaval, it is important to watch and listen carefully to what your teenager is doing and saying. Life today brings greater pressures and stresses, and many adolescents have difficulty handling them. Depressed adolescents are more likely to abuse drugs and alcohol, and suicide is a terrible possibility. Before the 1970s, teenage suicide was a rare event; now, nearly half a million teenagers attempt suicide each year. Since 1960, teenage suicides have doubled. Among

SIGNS OF DEPRESSION

Anyone who met Ted thought he had the world by the tail. The youngest of three athletically gifted brothers, Ted was a seventeen-year-old superstar. He played three varsity sports, excelled at competitive diving, and was a good student. His parents had been through the teen years with his brothers, so when Ted began withdrawing from them during his junior year, they initially chalked it up to teenage moodiness.

"The red flag for me was when I started noticing the change in the state of his room," explains his mother. "Ted was always a really orderly child. During his junior year, he started leaving his room in total disarray—and it wasn't just messy, it was dirty. This was something the Ted I knew would never have tolerated. We also joked about the fact that he was going through his 'black period'—wearing only black clothes and even keeping his room really dark, with all sorts of depressing posters on the walls. The most maddening thing was that Ted would have his friends over and seem just fine, joking with them and appearing to be happy; but, as soon as they left, he'd go back into his cave and refuse even to talk with us. The more we asked about how he was doing, the further he pulled away."

Fortunately, Ted had a good relationship with the male adolescent medicine doctor he and brothers saw and, when his mother made an extra appointment for him, he was willing to go. Talking to a man he trusted, Ted was able to open up and discuss the pressures he felt about his life—his many activities coupled with time-consuming homework assignments and tutoring for the SATs. When the doctor asked, Ted even admitted he occasionally wished it were "all over." He insisted that he'd never deliberately try to kill himself, "because of what that would do to my folks." Ted met with this doctor twice more—once with his parents, when they discussed what Ted could cut from his schedule. He also accepted a referral to a psychiatrist who put Ted on medication for a time and helped Ted come to terms with what he wanted out of life and what he thought was expected of him.

young people aged fifteen to nineteen, suicide is the second leading cause of death.

Many teenagers develop an intense interest in mortality and the drama of life. Most of the time, this is just a part of the maturation process. You should be cautiously alert to any major changes in your child's personality or interests. Many times, teenagers who have suicidal thoughts have experienced depression and are then faced with an acute crisis. Remember, though, that what they view as a crisis—the loss of a boyfriend or girlfriend, a run-in with a favorite teacher—may not be what you consider a big deal. Other important danger signs are the use of alcohol or other substances and isolation from peers and other support systems.

If your child exhibits obvious personality changes and threatens to "end it all" or begins to give away possessions, take action immediately. A suicide attempt results when a teenager is completely overwhelmed and unable to cope. Boys are four times more likely to kill themselves, but girls are three times more likely to attempt it.

Self-injury is another possible outlet for the depressed teenager. If you are worried that your child is feeling suicidal—especially if there have been any threats of self-harm—you can never be too cautious. Think about what you have in your house that could be used in a suicide attempt and remove the temptation, if possible. Guns are by far the most common items used in successful suicides. If you have a gun, even if you are sure your child doesn't know where it is, remove it from the home or secure it. Similarly, if you have large supply of medicines (acetaminophen, or Tylenol, is especially worrisome because it can destroy the liver), remove them.

Don't be afraid to talk to your child about your concerns. Evidence clearly shows that talking about suicide does not markedly increase the likelihood of a teenager attempting suicide. On the con-trary, it often defuses the situation, and can better inform you as to how worried you should be. If you're not sure, seek help from a suicide-prevention hotline, the pediatrician, a school counselor, or someone else who has experience in assessing suicide risk.

What Causes It?

Sometimes depression can result from what is simply "bad luck." If a child has lost a parent or grandparent, or if some other traumatic event has occurred in the child's life, it can bring on a depressive mood. However, two siblings may have shared common experiences, but often only one of them suffers a mood disorder as a result. Each child's reaction may result from many factors, including the age at the time of the incident and the child's emotional makeup. Some people are simply emotionally hardier than others. Depression also seems to have a genetic component. If a child is diagnosed with depression, it is likely that at least one parent or other close relative has also suffered from a mood disorder.

Much research over the past thirty years has focused on biological roots of depression. Advances in medications known to alleviate depression have led to a focus on two important brain neurotransmitters, norepinephrine and serotonin, as potential causes. These are the compounds that are supposedly out of balance when people talk about depression being the result of a "chemical imbalance." It is currently impossible to measure the amounts of these neurotransmitters in the human brain, so researchers either create animal models of depression to study or measure substances found in human blood or urine that may indirectly reflect the activity of these neurotransmitters. To date, neither approach has offered a convincing explanation of how depression affects brain function or how a change in brain function might cause depression.

Mania, too, is a mystery. Although related to depression, it is more than just its opposite. The great majority of people who are depressed never experience mania. Some patients can have severe, recurrent episodes of mania and never have episodes of depression. Again, researchers have pinpointed norepinephrine and serotonin, as well as another neurotransmitter, acetylcholine, as brain chemicals likely related to mania, but the evidence for their involvement remains weak.

It is important to note that essentially all of this research has been done in adults. Little to no progress has been made researching this disorder in those still developing. We know that the brain changes enormously from birth all the way into the early twenties. How those changes might affect the symptoms or even the causes of depression or mania still is a mystery.

Oftentimes, parents worry that they have somehow caused their child to be depressed. At times, life circumstances certainly play a central role. Major moves, divorces, and other life events are stressful, and stress increases the risk of bad reactions, including depression, especially in vulnerable individuals. However, depression also commonly occurs at random. Psychiatrists call this endogenous depression, and it is rare in children under age eight. After that age, it grows increasingly more common.

Rather than worry about the reasons why, parents need to focus on changes in behavior. It is crucial to know if your child is reacting to something in his environment. However, as with other disorders, depression is a complex interaction between individual biological and psychological vulnerabilities and environmental influences. It is less helpful to place blame and more important to recognize that your child is in trouble and needs help.

Serious consequences can result if mood disorders are ignored. The recurrence rate of untreated depression in children is about 50 percent. These children are less likely to do well in school, make friends, or become involved in extracurricular activities; as a result, self-esteem suffers and depression may deepen. Suicide is certainly one frightening potential result of unrecognized depression, but there are many others.

The Diagnosis

Diagnosing depression is not always easy. Much of the crucial information has to come from the individual, and many adolescents and younger children are either unaware of their feelings or unwilling to share them. Also, depression often occurs along with other conditions such as eating disorders, ADHD, substance abuse, or behavior problems, and parents and other responsible adults may simply not think about depression as a potential added or even causative problem.

Your job as a parent is not to diagnosis the disorder, but rather to recognize the possibility that there is something wrong. The professional's job is to look more deeply into your child's behavior and determine if depression might be present. Again, there is no conclusive laboratory test or brain scan to test for depression; we must rely on information gathered from the child, the family, and other significant figures, such as teachers.

Depression is an internalizing disorder, meaning that unlike ADHD, an externalizing disorder, most of its essential signs and symptoms occur inside the individual, and are not directly observable. As a result, diagnosis becomes much more dependent on the patient. Parents can, of course, provide invaluable information about changes in behavior, but only the child can talk about their mood, energy level, capacity for enjoyment, and suicidal thoughts or intentions.

Methods for gathering such information vary among professionals, and can also differ by the age of the patient. Some professionals use standardized questionnaires or inventories that address an array of common signs and symptoms of depression. They might use such an inventory as a part of a direct interview with the patient or have the patient fill it out independently (on paper or on a computer). Other professionals ask a similar range of questions without using a form. You might wonder if a child or adolescent would answer truthfully, but research shows that many do, and most such inventories have repeat or "trick" questions to make sure the answers are more than just random entries.

With very young children (under six or seven years old), depression is usually related to chaotic or abusive environments, so the main focus becomes gathering information about what is going on in the child's life. Few children that age have developed the ability to observe themselves, so it can be especially difficult to get direct statements about how they feel. Observing their play can often provide helpful information;

for example, a depressed child's play may seem especially listless, playing alone with creatures or dolls and not wanting to be around others much.

Projective tests, typically administered by trained psychologists, can also help diagnose depression in children. Common examples are the Rorschach inkblots and the Children's Apperception Test (CAT). The former, familiar to almost everyone, uses photographs of inkblots already administered to tens of thousands of individuals of all ages. The types of common responses are characterized by how they change during development (from childhood through adolescence into adulthood), and how they are affected by disorders such as depression. The CAT is less intimidating. It consists of a number of stimulus cards that depict a range of scenes, like a boy sitting on the floor looking at a violin that he is holding in his hand, and the child is asked to tell a story about each card. Like the Rorschach inkblots, responses to each card are compared to thousands of others. Just as the

MANIFESTATIONS OF DEPRESSION

Nicole, age eleven, was brought to my office because her parents thought she was depressed. Looking back, her parents realized that their daughter had always seemed gloomy. She always expected the worst—that rain would spoil her plans for an outdoor birthday party, that her favorite dress would get a stain that wouldn't come out, that her cat was getting old and would die soon. Still, she seemed to be doing fine all through elementary school. She had friends, did well academically, and was earnest and sensitive, just not especially happy. Then came middle school. At first, Nicole talked to her parents about some troubles she was having finding a group to be with at lunch and to walk with from class to class. But Nicole's parents worked and they had two other children—while they listened with concern, they assumed everything would smooth out as the year went on.

Nicole began sleeping much more than she used to, often taking a nap right after school and going to bed by 8:30 P.M. In addition, Nicole was eating much more and had gained weight, partly because she no longer did any kind of exercise. Her parents attributed these changes to the fact that Nicole had entered adolescence. Nicole's report card was the wake-up call: After earning As and Bs on her first middle school report card, by midyear, her grades had slipped. One teacher even sent home a note requesting a meeting with her parents. Understandably worried, Nicole's parents got a referral from their pediatrician and connected with a professional who specialized in cognitive therapy and was able to help with Nicole's depression.

pessimist is apt to see the darker possibilities of any situation, the depressed child typically tells stories that have bleaker themes and more negative outcomes.

As important as family information, questionnaires, and psychological tests can be, the ultimate diagnostic instrument is the mental health professional. He or she must take the cumulative data and synthesize it into a diagnosis that accurately describes what is happening to your child and what needs to be done about it.

Treatment

Depression is treatable, so if you suspect that your child is depressed, look for help. Most children with depression can be treated effectively with antidepressant medications, certain types of psychotherapy, or a combination of both. Treatment should begin with a full evaluation and an assessment to rule out any other underlying physical disease or illness that could also produce depression-like symptoms. The prognosis for successful treatment is good, and the potential consequence of not getting effective treatment can be severe.

Dysthymic Disorder

Dysthymic disorder is a less severe but more chronic form of depression that can have similar symptoms to those for de-

pression. While the depressive symptoms may be less overwhelming for the child, dysthymia is long-lasting and pervasive, and its effects can be quite profound.

What Is It?

Dysthymic disorder used to be called minor depression—or how parents sometimes describe "mopey kids." To be diagnosed with dysthymic disorder, a child need not exhibit as many symptoms as for major depression, but the symptoms must last longer (at least a year). As with adults, many of these children go through life always a little depressed and dysfunctional. However, they are at a markedly increased risk for developing a major depression that may overwhelm them for weeks to months, only to return to their dysthymic baseline. This vulnerability has led clinicians to be more proactive in identifying and treating these children. Even for those who don't experience major depression, the persistent low mood and energy level may deprive them of many valuable experiences they might otherwise enjoy.

The Diagnosis

Perhaps one of the most frustrating aspects of looking for depression in children is that the child himself may not know that the label applies to him. It is the rare child who comes to a parent saying, "I'm feeling really down right now, and I don't think this is normal." Instead, parents are likely to hear complaints about headaches or stomachaches, notice a general irritability, or a lack of energy or enthusiasm. If this is a chronic, persistent pattern, as occurs with dysthymia, parents might simply to come to view such behaviors as normal for that child.

There is little agreement about exactly how to diagnose dysthymia in a child. Quite often, these children don't even come to professional attention until they fall into a depression. Their baseline symptoms become apparent only as the mental health professional learns what the child was like before the major depression began. If you have a child with a low number of symptoms or mild severity, don't worry about trying to make a diagnosis. If you become concerned that such symptoms are really interfering with your child's ability to function at home, at school, or with friends, then it may be time to seek an evaluation. The assessment itself will be quite similar to that described for depression.

Treatment

Medications for dysthymic disorder have not been well documented and probably are not the optimal intervention. Cognitive therapy, however, can be effective. If children or adolescents can gain a better understanding of their condition and learn better coping methods, they may be able to avoid suffering from major depressions.

Bipolar Disorder

This disorder is distinguished by both emotional highs and lows—it is a true emotional roller coaster. Bipolar disorder differs from depression because patients also experience manic episodes or periods of extraordinary mood elevation.

CHANGING TIMES

When I started studying psychiatry in the mid-1970s, bipolar disorder was thought to be only an adult problem. By the mid-1980s, clinical researchers had convincingly shown that bipolar disorder could occur earlier, even as early as young teens, but was still thought to be rare. I recall a single case report published in 1984 of a four-and-a-half-year-old who was "silly" all the time, required only a few hours sleep each night, talked a mile a minute, and was so convinced he was Superman that he kept trying to jump off high surfaces to prove he could fly. It was published at the time precisely because it seemed such a rarity.

What Is It?
. . . .

Anyone who has spent time around children knows that a twelve-year-old girl can be giggling and laughing with friends in the afternoon and crying about a bad score on a math test later on that evening. This type of behavior is perfectly normal for children and teenagers who may arguably experience "higher highs" and "lower lows" than do adults, but who are also less adept at keeping their emotions in check. The most striking difference between younger patients and adults is that irritability is the most common emotion in children and adolescents rather than happiness or elation.

Bipolar disorder is different from these ups and downs both because the episodes are disabling and the emotional and behavioral symptoms are not closely linked to what is actually happening to the person. The child who is excited about going to Disneyland may be understandably giddy about the upcoming trip; the child suffering bipolar disorder may be hyper or irritable for no discernible reason and the happiness, silliness, or hyperactivity is likely to be completely out of sync with the moods of other children.

Bipolar disorder may begin with either manic or depressive symptoms. The depressions are impossible to distinguish from those described above, although people with bipolar disorder are more vulnerable to having psychotic depressions.

In addition to the symptoms of depression, additional symptoms of bipolar disorder may include:
- Severe changes in mood, particularly in relation to others of the same age and background. This can be unusually happy or silly, or very irritable, angry, agitated, or aggressive.
- Inflated sense of self-esteem, often a sense of invulnerability.
- Decreased need for sleep, sometimes only one to two hours, or even going without sleep at all and only incurring minimal fatigue.
- Significant increase in talkativeness, coupled with an inability to stay on topic.
- Major increase in activities, initially accompanied by an increase in productivity but followed by more and more partially completed tasks.
- Appearance of or a marked increase in sexual behavior, usually far more intense and with poorer social awareness than would be expected for the child's age. (The intensity of the sexual behavior often raises the question of sexual abuse, a possibility that must be considered.)
- High risk-taking behavior, such as drug or alcohol abuse, reckless driv-

ing, or sexual promiscuity, with the main ingredient being poor judgment.

One fourteen-year-old I treated for bipolar disorder came into my office that really gave me the sense of a person "bouncing off the walls." Talking at about triple the speed of an average person, he described to me how he was normally shy, but over the weekend he'd attended a party and for the first time ever stayed the whole time and made many friends. "Everyone loved me," he told me. He also happily showed me the list he'd made during the ten minutes spent in the waiting room, of fifty CDs that he had suddenly decided he had to have immediately—once he bought a CD player.

While being "up," having lots of energy, and feeling positively about oneself sounds good, it is all a matter of degree. As the mania grows more severe, the individual becomes increasingly flooded with ideas, plans, and desires. Judgment is impaired, often leading to impulsive spending, drug use, and sexual activity that can produce permanent damage. Hallucinations and delusions can occur. A patient's mood can go from happy to euphoric or irritable and impatient at the drop of a hat.

Children or teens with bipolar disorder are very difficult to be around. Their level of energy and intense emotional re-actions soon wear thin, and some of their ideas can be worrisome—it is difficult to safeguard someone who thinks he actually has superpowers. One patient was so convinced of his invulnerability that he wanted to stand in the middle of the street to see what damage would occur to a car running into him. Fortunately, he retained enough compassion for others to worry about what might happen to the driver of the car if he actually tried that particular experiment. Even more fortunately, his family realized his need for immediate help.

What Causes It?

Over the past fifteen years, interest in childhood-onset bipolar disorder has reached near fever pitch. For the past several years, more than half of the children I assess in a weekly consultation clinic have been referred to us to rule out bipolar disorder. In my opinion, few of them have that diagnosis, but some do.

What has changed is the perception that bipolar disorder may look different in children, especially before puberty, than it does in adults. Some researchers have argued that childhood-onset bipolar disorder is often a chronic problem rather than one that comes and goes. Instead of clear episodes of depression or mania, the child has a bit of both, a mixed state that mainly comes out as an irritable mood with rapid fluctuations from cheerful to angry to placid over the course of hours or even minutes. Sleep is sometimes disturbed but not necessarily shortened, and many exhibit signs and symptoms that overlap heavily with ADHD, including distractibility, impulsivity, and hyperactivity. Many also are oppositional and some show signs of severe anxiety.

Many mental health professionals have met these children and been baffled by them, and it is unclear whether asserting that they have bipolar disorder helps them or their parents. In my experience, as troubling and difficult as treating these children can be, they do not fit the descriptions for "classic" bipolar disorder. Furthermore, the limited longitudinal studies (repeated assessments of the same subjects over a number of years) available to date raise serious doubts about how many children with these symptoms actually go on to develop bipolar disorder later in life. Although it certainly would be possible to argue that they outgrow the problem, this is not typical with bipolar disorder in adults. The following description is a more conservative view of bipolar disorder in young patients than you might find elsewhere. I believe that the best research currently available affirms that bipolar disorder can occur in younger children, but it does so rarely until midadolescence.

The Diagnosis

Because this is a multifaceted disorder, a diagnosis can only be made after careful observation over an extended period of time. Children in the manic phase may resemble children with ADHD; however, bipolar children are typically only that driven when they are manic. Also, they tend to be more sexually preoccupied, more grandiose (believing they have abilities well above their actual skills), and need considerably less sleep.

When diagnosing bipolar disorder, a professional must first rule out other causes for the symptoms, such as substance abuse, a reaction to medication, another medical condition, or other behavioral disorders. Often, they will order tests to rule out the possibility of an overactive thyroid, seizures, or a brain tumor. Most of the time such tests come back within the normal range.

Standard questionnaires about common manic symptoms are available and may be part of a child's testing. Family history can be informative, because bipolar disorder has a genetic component. However, the presence or absence of bipolar disorder even in a mother or father is by no means definitive. Many adolescents with clearly defined bipolar disorder have no family history, and most children who have a parent with bipolar disorder do not develop bipolar disorder themselves.

As with depression, the diagnosis of bipolar disorder remains a clinical decision. Because of the implications this diagnosis can have, both about treatments to avoid and about treatments your child may need, it is especially important that it be made by a trained professional who works with children and has experience with this disorder. Because of the controversies in the field, you should weigh the doctor's evidence not just about the diagnosis but also about the treatment implications.

Treatment
. . . .

Treatment approaches for bipolar disorder include a growing class of medications called mood stabilizers. Antidepressants often play an important role in helping with the depressive part of the emotional pendulum. Psychotherapy helps the patient understand himself, adapt to stresses, rebuild self-esteem, and improve relationships.

Medications
For a child coping with depression, carefully prescribed medications can be extremely helpful. Before starting a medication, specific target symptoms should be identified in a discussion between parent, child, and professional, and possible side effects should be explained.

The most commonly prescribed antidepressants are a class of drugs called selective serotonin reuptake inhibitors (SSRIs). One of the first, fluoxetine, commonly known as Prozac, was also the first antidepressant that the FDA specifically endorsed for use in children and adolescents. Since the mid-1980s, a number of SSRIs have become available in the United States, and their use in children and adolescents has expanded markedly. Concerns have arisen in the past few years due to reports that a small percentage of children and adolescents (and probably adults) may become more suicidal shortly after they start taking an antidepressant—even if they have not been suicidal before. In my opinion, this current concern reflects a broader principle: There is no such thing as a completely safe medicine.

Hospitalization may be necessary for the seriously depressed child. If you are at all concerned about the possibility of your child hurting herself or others, consult with a professional. At the same time, do not be afraid to explore the possibility that your child might be thinking about hurting herself; asking will not suddenly make her decide to do so. On the contrary, children (especially those who are worried they really might do something) often find it relieving to have someone ask them the question.

THE DIFFERENCE BETWEEN DISORDERS

Until age eleven, Lisa was a wonderful child who gave her parents no problems. Then, abruptly, she became moody and withdrawn. Her grades went from As to Ds, and she began experimenting with a variety of unacceptable activities ranging from taking drugs to having unprotected sex. After an exceedingly difficult three years, life suddenly seemed to settle down for her. In fact, her parents were amazed. Although they worried that she was still a little wild, she became much sweeter with them, began to show renewed interest in school, and started reaching out to old friends; she seemed well on the road to recovery. She was bright enough that she quickly caught up with her studies. Midway through her sophomore year in high school, however, she began complaining that she felt fidgety and restless and had trouble concentrating at school. In contrast, her parents reported that sometimes she would be so excited about an assignment that she seemed to have boundless energy and enthusiasm, sometimes working far into the night. They decided to send Lisa for a battery of psychological testing; the tests showed Lisa to have marked problems with impulsivity and poor attention, and the psychologist suggested she be evaluated for ADHD.

By the time Lisa came to see me, she had grown increasingly irritable and suspicious of her parents' motives. She was sleeping only about two or three hours a night. Her energy remained high, as did her enthusiasm for various projects, but her ability to actually complete projects had dropped dramatically, and her performance in school was again suffering. Two days after I met Lisa and diagnosed her with bipolar disorder, she began hearing voices telling her how special she was. A brief hospitalization was necessary, because she had become convinced that her parents were actively trying to harm her because of her unique role in the world. Fortunately, she responded well to treatment and was able to return to a normal life after only a few months.

The use of antidepressants for treating depression in children and adolescents dates back to the late 1970s, and has been a source of both considerable excitement and substantial consternation. Studies that seemed to illustrate the benefits of antidepressants were part of the arguments used to persuade the field that even young children can suffer from depression. However, large-scale, well-designed studies that demonstrate a clear superiority of antidepressants over placebos for treating depressed children and adolescents are few, and the subject remains controversial.

What is clear is that antidepressants

do not affect the root cause of depression, whatever that may be. Relapse rates—that is, the likelihood that a child will again become depressed after stopping the antidepressant—are quite high. Because depression itself waxes and wanes, it may be possible to go for long periods without needing an antidepressant; however, each new episode of depression increases the likelihood that additional ones will occur. This often leads to patients who are doing well and have minimal side effects from the antidepressant simply staying on them indefinitely.

Nondrug Therapy

Therapy, with or without an antidepressant, can also be very helpful. Individual psychotherapy, for younger children, or play therapy, can encourage exploration of feelings and can help work through a sense of loss, powerlessness, or danger. Any illness during childhood or adolescence is likely to affect self-confidence—even as adults, most of us tend to think of ourselves as invulnerable until some trauma proves us wrong. A decrease in function due to a depressive or manic episode can seriously undermine a child's sense of self. In addition, since both depression and mania are recurring, it is important for the child to learn early signs that could indicate a return of symptoms. This, in turn, can facilitate early interventions.

Depressed children personalize failure and have difficulty finding positives in their lives, so cognitive behavioral therapy can help them deal with the irrational beliefs and distorted thoughts such as, "No one likes me!" or "I can never do anything right" that are part of depression. Group therapy and family therapy can also be beneficial. Working in a group can help children learn social skills and overcome a sense of solitude. Family therapy helps root out some of the issues that may have come about because of trouble within the family.

Other Ways to Help

As a parent of a child who is depressed or manic, your first and most important task is to take him seriously. Don't be dismissive of his feelings, or make comments like, "Oh, cheer up. Things can't be that bad." Moreover, don't assume that you know what he means. "I could just kill myself" is far more often an expression of frustration than a cry for help. But if it is the latter, you want to know.

You also don't want to encourage a child to wallow in their sadness, so you should try to find a balance: Acknowledge that he or she is having a rough time, but don't grow so distraught yourself that the child panics. Emphasize that you want to know what is going on and that you want to help. Reassure your child that other children feel this way too, and that it can get better. Ask the child if he feels safe and, if not, what he needs to feel safer.

Here are some simple things that help everyone feel better:

- Moderate aerobic exercise has been shown to relieve depressive symptoms in almost half of young adults.
- Good sleeping and eating habits can also help alleviate symptoms.
- Participation in enjoyable activities or ones that prove the child's self-worth improve mood and sense of self. Imaging studies show that altruistic behavior lights up the brain's reward areas.

The depressed or manic child is, for the most part, incapable of problem-solving. While there is no substitute for professional help, one thing parents can do is model behavior that provides strategies for keeping life in control. For example, if your ten-year-old is depressed and having trouble getting through her homework, sit down with her after school or when you get home from work, and make a list together of everything she must do that evening. (Eventually, you can encourage her to create this list as she goes through the school day.) Long-term assignments should be broken down into small parts that can be done each day.

When a child is having a tough time, he or she may understandably require extra attention. This may mean sitting with your son and paying bills while he does his homework, or canceling your Saturday night plans when you discover your fifteen-year-old is going to be all alone and isn't happy about it.

The Bottom Line

While a put-on-a-happy-face attitude cannot solve the problems of a depressed child, you can continue to model a can-do approach to life. Therapy and possibly medication may be necessary, but it's also important to demonstrate the ability to control your surroundings by teaching them what to do to make things better. If friends leave your daughter out of their plans to go to a movie on Friday night, what fun thing can she think of to do? Is there another friend who might like to come over, or would she like to go over to her cousin's? With or without depression, the teen years can be tough; if your child is going through a difficult time, it is important that you be there to support her.

Chapter 6

Anxiety Disorders and Sleep Problems

At age nine, Laurie was having trouble in school. In November, her teacher called Laurie's parents to come in for a conference to discuss her concerns. "Laurie's fear of being in front of the class has really gotten out of hand," said the teacher. "We read aloud every day after lunch, and from the moment she enters the classroom in the afternoon, she is edgy and teary. Her face is flushed, and she usually asks to go to the bathroom while we're reading to avoid the possibility of being called on. She's missing so much of our class time that if we don't help her with this, she simply won't be able to keep up."

Tim's third-grade classmates couldn't wait until the May field trip to the zoo, but for Tim, the forthcoming excursion created almost unbearable anxiety. Tim suffered from a phobia of elephants since his parents took him to his first circus at age four, and the thought of seeing an elephant, even from far away, was terrifying to him. From the day the field trip was announced in early April, Tim went to bed fretting about what could happen to him. Every morning, Tim pleaded with his mother to let him skip the field trip.

At 9:15 P.M. when it was time for Diana's lights to be turned out, her dad always peeked in to say good night. Over time, her father noticed that Diana was rarely in bed at that time because her increasingly elaborate bedtime routine was growing longer and longer. Diana had to put everything on her homework desk "just so," straighten all the stuffed animals, and carefully fold each item of clothing she planned to wear the next day. If her dad spoke to her in the midst of this process, she would shriek at him, "Now I have to do everything ALL OVER again." And she would go back and re-straighten each thing she had previously touched.

Each of these children suffers from some form of anxiety disorder. Whether they are phobic, as Tim and Laurie are, or obsessive-compulsive, as Diana is, they are suffering from excessive and unnecessary anxiety, and they can be helped.

Anxiety disorders range from phobias and obsessive-compulsive disorder to generalized anxiety, separation anxiety, panic attacks, and post-traumatic stress disorder (PTSD). All anxiety disorders have in common a state of being excessively ill at ease, as one might feel when in danger or in an unfamiliar or particularly challenging situation. Children with anxiety disorders, however, have these feelings without a particular external cause or far in excess of a reasonable reaction. In addition, those suffering from an anxiety disorder may commonly complain of stomachaches, diarrhea, and fatigue. They may also feel on edge or be prone to angry outbursts.

As with adults, if a child were to be anxious for a day or two, or even a couple of weeks because of something happening in his life, it would not be a cause for alarm. Anxiety is classified as a disorder when it persists for a prolonged period of time or becomes so severe it hampers the child's ability to live a normal life and participate in sports, school, or family and social interactions.

Anxiety disorders can range from mild to severe. In children, these disorders are likely to become more pronounced at the beginning and end of the school years, when all children are likely to be a bit apprehensive. Other periods of heightened risk include external changes such as a major move, increased family tensions such as marital problems, or the arrival of a new baby.

LIVING WITH AN ANXIOUS CHILD

As with many aspects of parenting, dealing with a child who has an anxiety disorder is not something most parents plan on. If your child is anxious, you have probably experienced a range of emotions from sympathy and concern, to impatience and embarrassment. If your child has panic attacks, you may have rushed to an emergency room, fearful for her life, only to learn there's nothing really wrong. If your child has severe obsessions, you may have wondered if he could be crazy because he does the same thing over and over. You may have grown tired and impatient fearing that a suggestion of a change in activity will set off a tantrum. You may worry that life is passing your child by because she is so fearful of interactions with peers and never participates in class. Above all, you may vacillate between telling yourself there really is something wrong and scolding yourself for worrying over nothing.

If your child's behavior is impairing the ability for him or her to function, it is definitely not nothing. It's OK to seek help—both you and your child will feel better.

Most research shows timidity and nervousness, traits that are likely to lead to heightened anxiety, are inborn. In addition, if a child is born into a family with anxious parents, the behavior is nurtured. There is also strong evidence to suggest that environment contributes to anxiety both immediately (being in a high-stress situation where there is real or perceived risk), and over time (having been exposed to highly stressful situations in the past). One example of the latter comes from research on post-traumatic stress disorder, an especially severe response to witnessing or experiencing major trauma. Studies of Vietnam veterans who underwent torture and other horrors of war addressed why some developed PTSD and others did not. One powerful factor was the fact that those who had experienced a major trauma as children were at notably greater risk for PTSD than were those who had not. This suggested that the early trauma may have sensitized those individuals so their response to a later trauma was more severe.

Exactly what happens in the brain to cause anxiety disorders is still not fully understood, although considerable research has emerged over the past decade. Attention to potential dangers is a very basic survival mechanism—even primitive single-cell organisms recognize and respond to danger by moving away from it. Some of the most primitive parts of the brain monitor input from both the whole body and from the newer parts of the brain where thinking is believed to occur. When danger threatens, those systems rapidly assess the nature and severity of the risk. If the danger seems serious, they set a series of reactions into motion that prepare the body to either fight or flee. It seems likely that various factors, ranging from genetic to past experience to psychological, can alter the threshold at which these systems perceive danger. A sense of being at risk, then, can compound the problem, creating a spiral that proves disabling for a surprisingly large percentage of the general population.

The following is a breakdown of the types of anxiety disorders commonly seen in children and adolescents.

Generalized Anxiety Disorder

Generalized anxiety disorder (GAD) is characterized by a prolonged period (at least several months) of chronic, exaggerated worry and tension that is more severe than most people experience.

What Is It?

According to her parents, Missy had been a worrier all her life. As a baby, she was exceptionally unwilling to let anyone but her mother hold her. Her father joked that even he was scarcely acceptable most of the time. She never liked change. Picking her up from preschool was almost as difficult as dropping her off. She reacted poorly to new clothes and almost always had to have the inner labels cut off. She also had a narrow range of foods she would eat.

Once she started elementary school, her parents dreaded the beginning of each school year. Until Missy, who was a bright and winsome child, became comfortable with her teachers, she made their lives miserable. Despite all these issues, the family did not even consider seeking help until they suddenly had to move across the country because of a job transfer. That move, along with her father spending considerably less time with the family, was simply too much for eight-year-old Missy. She began to worry that something bad would happen to her parents, she couldn't focus on her work at school, and often was tearful and afraid, even at home with her parents. This was what finally brought them to my office.

Nan's anxiety began under perfectly normal circumstances. It was her junior year of high school, and she was taking five advanced-placement classes, playing a starting position on the field hockey team, and preparing to take the SATs in the spring. Her parents brought her to me in early June. They had tolerated her anxiety until after the SATs were over. However, her emotional state failed to improve, and she got to the point where she could hardly make a decision without second-guessing herself and lashing out at friends and family. "We just felt like her anxiety was no longer in the 'understandable' range," said her mother.

When children suffer from GAD, they worry about many things, large and small. A child may invest the same amount of worry over an upcoming quiz as he will about a beloved grandparent who has been hospitalized. These children will also exhibit random feelings of anxiety. Headaches, stomachaches, muscle aches, diarrhea, irritability, and difficulty sleeping can all be symptoms of generalized anxiety disorder. Frequent visits to the school nurse may also be a sign that a child is unable to stop worrying.

What Causes It?

About 3 to 4 percent of the U.S. population suffers from generalized anxiety disorder, and it seems to run in families. The disorder usually starts in childhood or adolescence, and affects more girls than boys. Symptoms usually start slowly and build over time to the point that the child or the family realizes that help is needed. To complicate matters, GAD often co-exists with depression or other anxiety-related issues.

THE EFFECTS OF ANXIETY

For Marian, the problem manifested itself first with sleepovers. Since the beginning of fourth grade, she and her best friend, Tricia, had alternated homes for sleepovers almost every week. At Marian's house they loved popping popcorn and curling up on the sofa to watch movies before being ushered off to bed by Marian's parents. At Tricia's, the attraction was her grandmother who frequently babysat for the family on Friday nights. Tricia's grandmother never tired of board games and Tricia, Marian, and Tricia's little brother, Josh, played everything they could until it was time for bed.

One night, Tricia and Marian had a wonderful time playing hide-and-seek around the house with Tricia's brother, and they had concluded the evening with a game with Tricia's grandmother. At bedtime, Marian became teary, and within a half an hour was crying inconsolably. Tricia's grandmother suggested Marian call her parents, and though that reassured her temporarily, by 11:15 P.M. Marian was again unable to cope with her overwhelming emotions. At 11:30 P.M. the grandmother placed another call to the parents to pick Marian up.

The next week, the girls went to Marian's home for a sleepover as usual. They had a great time, but the following week Marian backed out of going to Tricia's. Tricia then came to Marian's for a couple of weeks in a row, but the change in their routine—and Tricia's desire for the special evenings with her grandmother—soon brought an end to the sleepover tradition the girls shared. While their friendship at school continued, Tricia made other friends who were more flexible about playdates and sleepovers.

While it was easy enough for Marian's parents to accommodate Marian's desire to forego sleepovers, Marian was starting to have other issues. Marian had started balking when it was time to go to school. Although by October she had only missed a day or two of class, her parents were no longer able to handle the stress of cajoling ten-year-old Marian to get dressed and ready for school. They were ready for professional help.

Any parent who has left a crying two- or three-year-old at daycare will recognize the signs of separation anxiety. What makes Marian's case notable is that her anxiety is not age-appropriate. The fact that her anxiety occurred in a home where she had formerly been very comfortable, and that it prevented her from doing something she wanted to do, was extremely troubling.

At first, Marian's parents simply helped her avoid the situation, assuming that this was a phase that would pass. When they approached me the following fall, they told me that they had hit their stress limit because they were spending so much time every day trying to get Marian out of the house and to school on time.

The Diagnosis

As with other psychiatric disorders, a diagnosis of GAD rests upon information gathered from the child, parents, and other involved adults. In this instance, the clinician is looking for a pattern of fearful responses and excessive levels of worry or concern that characterize a child's functioning in most settings. There are a few standardized questionnaires that the clinician may ask adults to complete about the child, or teenagers to fill out about themselves; but they are used to ensure that the evaluation covers a variety of fears and the situations in which they occur.

In many ways, GAD is the simplified model of anxiety. Rather than having a specific, focused fear or obsession, the child is worried about virtually everything. The most important task for a clinician is to confirm that there is no real basis for the worries (abuse, trauma, concealed family conflicts) or that they don't stem from another psychiatric source, such as the beginnings of a psychosis.

Treatment

Once diagnosed, GAD is very treatable with psychotherapy, medications, or a combination of both. For a more complete discussion, see the end of this chapter.

Separation Anxiety Disorder

Separation anxiety is a normal stage of childhood. It only becomes a disorder if a child does not outgrow it or if it becomes so severe and pervasive that it interferes with the child's and parents' ability to function normally.

What Is It?

Separation anxiety is a normal part of child development. Stranger anxiety surfaces in babies as young as six months who become alarmed if held by someone who is unfamiliar to them. By about eleven to twelve months, babies may still be fearful, but they begin to understand that the stranger who tickles their tummy isn't going to grab them away from their mom's loving arms. Between eighteen months and three years, separation anxiety is also normal. While some two-year-olds can walk into a classroom with no problem, the majority will be hesitant for a few days, and some will be quite clingy; this is all perfectly normal.

Separation anxiety becomes a problem when it persists in children age four and above; approximately 96 percent of young children can successfully separate at this stage. A new sibling or some other change in the family may make even a four-year-old clingy for a while, but the phase should pass relatively quickly. And while thirty five-year-olds invited to a playground for a birthday party will run off and start playing, two or three perfectly normal children will be reluctant to have their parents leave them. Tommy or Theresa may look around and see a frantic hostess, an overwhelmed babysitter, and a man in a clown suit, all trying to bring control to a large number of children; their inability to separate in this circumstance should not be judged as pathological. We, as parents, might think this party doesn't look like much fun either.

The older child who suffers from separation anxiety may have headaches, stomachaches, diarrhea, dizziness, rapid heartbeat, and other physical manifestations of discomfort. They are also usually preoccupied with thoughts that something bad is going to happen to them or their parents if they are separated. Because the child's intent is to remain connected to the parent and not to leave home, separation anxiety is sometimes first diagnosed as a school phobia.

Children do need to attend school, and it might even be considered a psychological "emergency" when they don't. School is an ongoing and socially active world, and the child who is absent frequently begins to suffer both socially and academically. The combination of the initial separation anxiety coupled with the issues that result from falling behind in school, may make a child even more anxious. If at all possible, the child needs to continue going to school and maintaining a normal routine.

What Causes It?

Both separation anxiety and panic disorders are related to a defect in the way that the brain recognizes and responds to danger. These children's bodies are releasing norepinephrine, a chemical our bodies produce to respond to danger, at a time when there is no real danger. Children who suffer from separation anxiety may go on to suffer from panic attacks as adolescents or adults (although panic attacks can occur with any type of anxiety).

Because there is a genetic component to this disorder, one parent may have also suffered something similar as a child. With all good intentions, they may make the situation worse by being overly sympathetic and "babying" the child in such a way that the child comes to believe that there is something about sleepovers, sleepaway camp, or school that is to be feared.

The Diagnosis

Separation anxiety can range from mild to severe, and can be disruptive to a child's life. If treated, however, the prognosis is quite good. Untreated, it may lead to chronic anxiety and persistent problems with school anxiety.

Like GAD, diagnosing separation disorder is largely a matter of confirming that the symptoms are present and that they are impairing a child's function. Then, a good clinician will work with you to rule out other possible explanations. For example, a child might temporarily be worried about leaving a parent who only recently recovered from a serious illness, or might be reacting to the stress of moving to a new home or starting a new school.

Treatment

Psychotherapy and medication can be quite helpful in treating separation anxiety, and these will be addressed in greater detail at the end of this chapter.

Phobias

A phobia is defined as an exaggerated and inexplicable fear that focuses on a specific object or situation.

What Is It?

We all know people with phobias. Fear of flying is a perfect example of how irrational thoughts trump rational ones in someone who is phobic. Despite statistics proving that airplane travel is far safer than driving, adults who fear flying refuse to do so and will convolute their personal and work lives so they never have to travel anywhere they can't drive.

The reality-TV program *Fear Factor* plays off the fact that people are "phobic" about certain things, and contestants are asked to do things like eat spiders and worms, drop from great heights on a zip line, or be in a room filled with snakes. Some people, like *Fear Factor* contestants, get giddy when facing their fears—and then go right ahead and confront it. Other people are essentially immobilized because of their fears. As with any of the anxiety disorders, when a child must alter the way he lives because of a fear, then it's time to address the issue.

Simple phobias, like fear of snakes, spiders, bees, dogs, heights, or tight spaces, are almost universal. The list of fears is nearly endless, and few people can declare truthfully that absolutely nothing makes them wary or fearful. But what if one of these fears become a major obstacle? What if, for example, a child is so fearful of snakes that even a picture of one produces such a reaction that parents must screen every book and magazine to which the child might have access? What if the child refuses to go to sleep each night until both parents spent an hour thoroughly checking the bedroom for spiders?

A SAMPLING OF PHOBIAS

achluophobia	fear of darkness	**hematophobia**	fear of blood
acousticophobia	fear of noise	**keraunophobia**	fear of thunder
acrophobia	fear of heights	**laliophobia**	fear of speaking
ailurophobia	fear of cats	**monophobia**	fear of being alone
aphephobia	fear of touching or being touched	**neophobia**	fear of anything new
arachnophobia	fear of spiders	**ophthalmophobia**	fear of being stared at
aviatophobia	fear of flying	**photophobia**	fear of light
claustrophobia	fear of confined spaces	**pyrophobia**	fear of fire
cynophobia	fear of dogs	**scoleciphobia**	fear of worms
dromophobia	fear of crossing streets	**sitophobia**	fear of food
emetophobia	fear of vomiting	**triskaidekaphobia**	fear of the number 13
enetophobia	fear of needles	**zoophobia**	fear of animals
graphophobia	fear of writing		

Being phobic or having irrational fears affects approximately 6.3 million Americans, and girls are more likely to have phobias than boys. Phobias usually first appear in childhood and adolescence, and are seen in about 2 percent of eleven-year-olds and approximately 5 percent of fourteen- to sixteen-year-olds.

What Causes It?

Sometimes understanding the cause of the phobia can lead to a solution. The parents of four-year-old Jeff came to see me because he had become phobic about mice and was refusing to go into his room for fear that one was in there. Initially, the parents were unsure about why Jeff had this particular fear. However, further discussion revealed that the fear developed immediately after an incident when Jeff's mother, who is terrified of mice, saw one in the hallway. According to the father, "When my wife saw that mouse, she screamed and climbed up on a chair, just like in a cartoon. With all the commotion, the mouse disappeared quickly, but she screamed for several minutes afterward." The child was a silent observer of the whole event, but the parents had not considered how he might interpret what had happened. Clearly, the mother's reaction to the presence of a mouse had left a considerable impression on their son.

Understanding that parent modeling had caused the phobia made it easier to treat it. In this case, the first step toward a solution was helping the parents see what had happened and encouraging them to talk about it with Jeff. His mother explained that she was scared of mice even though she knew they couldn't hurt anyone; his father said he wasn't scared of mice and even used to have one as a pet. In this instance, that was enough to relieve the fear and allow the child to go back into his bedroom, initially with the father as a protector.

Unfortunately, other phobias often grow from a complex series of fears and anxieties and are not nearly as simple to explain. Complex phobias involve much larger categories of situations or multiple phobias, so the individual has many more situations that must be avoided. For example, at age four, Geraldine had the fairly common problem of being afraid of the dark. Initially, this was easily managed with a nightlight in her room. However, after seeing the movie *Monsters, Inc.*, she began to fear that a monster was in her room and would insist that the parents check in the closet and under the bed. Then she became unable to go to bed by herself, insisting that one of her parents stay with her until she fell asleep. Soon even that was not enough. She would wake up at least once a night and demand to sleep in her parents' room.

By the time the family sought help, Geraldine's father had been sleeping on the floor in the child's room every night for several months. However, the reason the parents gave for coming to see me had nothing to do with night fears. It was only when their daughter began to insist that she could not be in a room alone, to the point that her mother could not even go to the bathroom by herself. Geraldine had to be in the bathroom with her or leave the door open, otherwise, she would stand at the door crying inconsolably.

The Diagnosis

Diagnosing a phobia is seldom a problem. Typically, the child or parent knows what the object of the fear is, and one or both can tell the clinician if the fear is problematic. Sometimes the fear is quite reasonable; for example, a child with a severe allergic reaction to bee stings may have a phobia of bees. Even then, if every buzzing noise causes the child to dissolve into tears, he may need help distinguishing between reasonable and excessive fear. In teenagers, the sudden emergence of an odd or unusual fear (for example, persistent concern that food or water might be contaminated or poisoned) may be an early sign of an emerging psychosis. It is important for the clinician to insure that, except for the specific fear, the patient is not having other problems with reality.

Treatment

Helping a child overcome a phobia can sometimes be easy. Four-year-old Sarah was terrified of dogs and refused to be in homes that had them. Her family decided getting a pet was one way to teach Sarah that dogs can be a positive force within a family. When she was five, Sarah's parents brought home a puffball of a puppy and introduced the dog to her very slowly. As Sarah became accustomed to the way the animal moved and responded, she grew more comfortable with all dogs. (Recently, Sarah announced to her family

that she was afraid of cats, but they have not yet decided to add a cat to the family.) Other phobias in children can often be worked through with psychotherapy and behavioral therapy, and in more difficult cases, medication.

Social Phobias

By far the most common of the anxiety disorders, a social phobia is an intense fear of becoming humiliated in social situations.

What Is It?

William, a sixteen-year-old concert-level violinist, loved playing and took pride in his musical skills. However, playing in public was becoming nearly impossible. Even thinking about a performance made him uneasy. Sometimes he would become physically ill during rehearsals, and he always felt sick before a performance. In addition, he found himself becoming increasingly shy around others, particularly those his own age. He was sure they knew his problem and would make fun of him.

Social anxiety has only recently been taken seriously. The fact that some people don't like to give speeches was never viewed as a disorder to be treated. However, this attitude is beginning to change, and people are realizing that speaking in front of others may not get any easier as you get older. For both children and adults, feeling nervous, nauseous, and having difficulty sleeping the night before a presentation is quite uncomfortable. And on the day of the presentation, the sweaty palms, racing heart, and flushed cheeks hardly help make a good impression.

While a social phobia is commonly discovered when a child is afraid to give a book report or an adult is nervous about delivering a speech, children with a social phobia also may express other fears, such as being afraid to enter a classroom late because everyone else will be watching, or eating lunch with others because they don't want other people to watch them eat.

What Causes It?

Today, approximately 5.3 million Americans suffer from social phobias. Those who suffer social phobias feel that others are more competent than they are. There may be a genetic component to this type of anxiety, and it may be accompanied by depression or other anxiety disorders. It usually begins in childhood or early adolescence, and it affects men and women equally. Although some individuals may associate the beginning of their fear with a specific event, it is more commonly a lifelong concern that waxes and wanes over time.

Treatment

While medication may eventually be helpful, psychotherapy and behavior modification should be the first approach for treating social fears. Educational and exposure interventions have proven beneficial by helping to normalize the feared experience. They also make the child

---

SELECTIVE MUTISM

One variant of social phobias seen especially in younger children is a disorder called selective mutism (formerly called elective mutism). Children with this disorder exhibit a partial to complete failure to speak in certain settings. To qualify for this diagnosis, children must be of normal intelligence and have normal language capabilities. In some situations (usually at home with their family) they seem perfectly fine. In other settings, like the classroom, they simply will not talk. This condition seems related to shyness, and many children grow out of it spontaneously. However, the longer selective mutism persists, the less likely it is to go away on its own. If you have a child who is more than eight or nine years of age with this problem and have not sought professional help, you should consider doing so.

aware that many other children have similar fears. Teaching coping techniques help increase self-confidence and, by gradually exposing the child to increasingly stressful situations, may help overcome the fear.

Panic Disorder

Panic disorder is manifested in panic attacks, brief but intense feelings of fear or terror that comes without warning and for no obvious reason. The symptoms are powerful enough that children and adults alike often become even more fearful because they don't know what is happening to them.

What Is It?

Having a panic attack is far more intense than simply feeling anxious or stressed out. The person having a panic attack may feel the world is spinning, or may become dizzy to the point of falling; overall, the physical sensations (racing heart, sweaty palms, difficulty breathing, tingling sensations, nausea, etc.) are so intense they can be quite frightening. Frequently, people experiencing a panic attack worry their hearts will burst or that they might die from lack of oxygen. The symptoms usually pass within ten minutes.

It can be difficult to recognize when

LIVING WITH A CHILD WITH PANIC DISORDER

Jonathan, a highly intelligent six-year-old, was generally anxious and hated unexpected events. His parents were never sure what would set him off and went to extraordinary lengths to make sure that he knew about family plans and other events that might upset him. One Saturday morning, his mother mentioned that a man was coming to wash all the windows of their house, including those in his room. Jonathan, startled, asked when. His mother told him that she wasn't sure but probably in a few hours. Jonathan began violently shaking his head no and his breathing rapidly increasing. Soon, he was screaming, "No, no, no," over and over as he raced between the two windows in his room, looking for the man. He continued this for twenty minutes, his concerned mother completely unable to offer consolation. Finally, he collapsed in his favorite hiding place, his closet, where he cuddled with a favorite blanket, mumbling, "Don't let the man come," until he finally fell asleep, exhausted. When he awoke, a half hour later, his mood had returned to normal, and he was actually excited about being able to watch the man wash the windows.

children are having panic attacks because they can't always convey exactly what they are experiencing. Adults who suffer panic attacks may go to the emergency room, fearing they are having a heart attack. Children, too, are often taken to the doctor because of the frightening symptoms. Some children in the midst of a panic attack may also become very angry—yet another obstacle to a correct diagnosis.

Unfortunately, panic disorder can be very debilitating. Victims of these attacks cannot tell when one may occur, and they often develop an intense fear of having them. For example, if your child has a panic attack at baseball practice, she may become very resistant to attending again. Sometimes children and adults can become agoraphobic because they become so intent on avoiding a panic attack.

What Causes It?

Panic disorder appears to be genetically based, and it affects women more than men. The exact mechanism by which a panic attack occurs is still poorly understood. Attacks can be precipitated (in those vulnerable) by fairly minor changes in the body's chemistry, but it is unclear if that is related to their cause or simply reflects the extraordinary sensitivity and awareness these individuals have for their body's functions.

The Diagnosis

Diagnosing a panic attack is primarily a matter of excluding other possible causes. These are primarily physical disorders, such as heart attack, certain rare tumors, low blood sugar (hypoglycemia), or excessive thyroid activity (hyperthyroidism). Similar symptoms can also occur with some drugs, such as large amounts of caffeine or stimulants. Panic attacks differ from generalized anxiety because they occur as discrete and brief events, with a clear beginning and end, whereas GAD is chronic.

Treatment

While panic attacks are quite frightening, this disorder is highly treatable. Treating panic disorder is especially important because a panic attack is a powerful motivator for change: In severe cases, untreated patients can become completely housebound, terrified that they will die or lose control if they leave. As with social phobias, education and exposure interventions can be helpful. There are also several medications that are effective at both shortening the panic attacks themselves and preventing panic attacks from occurring.

Obsessive-Compulsive Disorder

A child suffering obsessive-compulsive disorder (OCD) is plagued by persistent, recurring thoughts (obsessions like "I can't get clean!") usually accompanied by strong urges to perform specific actions (compulsions like repeated hand washing). Strikingly, even very young children with this disorder almost always know that both the thoughts and the actions are not sensible, but that makes them no less compelling.

What Is It?

OCD can occur in children as young as three years old. Of all the anxiety-type disorders, this is usually the easiest to recognize because the rituals to try to stop the anxious thoughts are often evident and elaborate—anything from the obsessive asking of questions to counting each stair in the staircase—and need to be started over if interrupted. Common fears that initiate the cycle of compulsive behavior include fear of contamination, persistent doubts about turning things off, or even aggressive impulses such as the urge to yell "Fire!" in a crowded theater.

Ritualized activities are incorporated into the person's daily routine and are not always directly related to the obsessive thought. **Some of the most common compulsions are:**

- **Cleaning**—a concern with germs and contamination that leads to obsessive washing, showering, or even cleaning the home
- **Checking**—checking that doors are locked or the stove is off (commonly adult activities)
- **Repeating**—usually actions, names, or phrases
- **Slowness**—an excessively slow and methodical approach to daily activities, with hours spent organizing and arranging objects
- **Hoarding**—an inability to throw away useless items, such as old newspapers, junk mail, even broken appliances, sometimes to the point where whole rooms are filled

Responsible people may check the stove more than once before leaving the house or drive back to double-check that they closed the garage door, but people with OCD may spend an hour or more a day performing these obsessive rituals. If OCD becomes severe enough, it can interfere with the normal pace of everyday life.

What Causes It?

OCD tends to run in families, and those

LIVING WITH A CHILD WITH OCD

June began worrying about getting dirty at about age eight, but could not exactly explain her concern to her parents. She first began having concerns about the bathrooms at school; at first it was all right for her to use the school bathrooms if she washed her hands both before and after going to the toilet and making sure the toilet seat was clean. Soon, she had to actually clean the toilet before using it, and eventually she learned to use the toilet without sitting down all the way. Despite all these precautions, she had to wash her hands thoroughly before and after each time This process gradually took longer and longer, until teachers complained about how much time June spent in the bathroom. After a few months, it simply became easier not to use the school toilets, because she did not have similar concerns about her toilet at home. Since her home was close to school, she found she could make it through the day by going to the bathroom there during the lunch hour.

June's fears gradually expanded and began to occur at home as well as at school. She began to worry that actually touching herself after using the toilet would make her so dirty no amount of hand washing could correct. She started stripping before using the toilet and then taking a shower afterward, sometimes, three to four a day, to avoid touching herself. By age ten, even that was not enough. She needed someone's help to make sure she was clean and talked her mother into taking a shower with her. Her mother reluctantly agreed when she could, because June was so heartbroken if she refused.

When June began to refuse to use her hands in the kitchen, her family finally, and with great reluctance, sought help. June had become so worried about getting dirty that she would not use her hands to touch surfaces that others had touched, opened the refrigerator with her shoulder, and opened and shut the fruit drawers with her feet. When that wouldn't work, she would demand that someone else get what she wanted.

who suffer from it may have other anxiety disorders as well. In the U.S., about 1 million children and teenagers, both boys and girls, have OCD—about one in every two hundred.

Over the past twenty years, a great deal of information about OCD has come to light, but its cause is still not completely understood. It seems to result from a defect in the interchange of signals between the front part of the brain cortex, where we process information, and some structures in the more primitive and basic part of the brain that help us sort out important information. Increasing serotonin activity in that part of the brain can markedly alleviate many of the symptoms, but that does not mean that OCD results from having too little serotonin. As with so much about brain function, there is still a lot to learn.

The Diagnosis

To diagnose OCD, the obsessions and compulsions need to take up considerable amounts of time—at least one hour per day—and interfere with normal routines. OCD can interfere with the ability to concentrate and it is not uncommon for a sufferer to avoid certain situations (for example, a person obsessed with cleanliness may avoid public restrooms). In addition, the individual must view these rituals as intrusive and unpleasant. In my experience, even children as young as four years old know their thoughts and actions are abnormal and would like to get rid of them. With teenagers, the clinician must also look for possible emerging psychoses, which sometimes accompany compulsive behaviors the child is using in an attempt to remain healthy.

There are several standardized questionnaires that some clinicians use to quantify the specific obsessions and compulsions a patient has, as well as their severity. Such instruments can be useful in monitoring progress over time.

Treatment

Cognitive therapy and medications are very helpful with OCD. The goal is to lessen the intensity of the anxious thoughts in order to reduce the need for the rituals. There are medications used to treat OCD, but their discontinuation is followed by as much as a 70 percent relapse rate. Cognitive therapy, however, appears to be more beneficial in helping the individual ward off the return of the disorder. Interestingly, brain scans of successfully treated individuals show that cognitive therapy and medications produce similar changes in the brain regions thought to be the site of this disorder.

Post-Traumatic Stress Disorder

Post-traumatic stress disorder (PTSD) is a debilitating emotional condition that develops following terrifying events. If stress symptoms last more than a month, then it is diagnosed as a disorder.

What Is It?

The general public first became familiar with post-traumatic stress disorder when soldiers returned from the Vietnam War began suffering horrifying daytime flashbacks, nightmares, and often acting out uncharacteristically because of the trauma they had experienced. However, you do not have to fight in a battle to suffer from PTSD.

Symptoms of PTSD include intrusive daytime thoughts about the trauma, nightmares, and sleep problems. Irritability, aggressiveness, acting inappropriate to age, or overreacting may also be present. While these symptoms can arise without an apparent cause, this disorder is sometimes set off by a particular trigger, such as an anniversary or physical reminder of the experience. (For example, if the trauma was seeing someone commit suicide by jumping out of a window, being on a high floor of a building might cause PTSD symptoms.)

PTSD occurs in 15 to 20 percent of children and adolescents who are exposed to severe trauma. Of course, exposure to traumatic events varies markedly across different settings, but no one is completely exempt. PTSD can inflict damage on a child's emotional development and ability to become independent, and is often accompanied by depression, substance abuse, or another anxiety disorder.

What Causes It?

Any type of catastrophic event a child may experience can cause PTSD—a life-threatening illness, severe injury, surviving abuse, or even a natural disaster. The devastating events of September 11, 2001, and Hurricane Katrina left both adults and children struggling with the emotional impact.

Emerging evidence, mainly from studies in adults, suggests that severe trauma may flood the brain with stress hormones, producing potentially permanent changes in future sensitivity to stress. As mentioned above, there is also good evidence that one risk factor for PTSD in adults is experiencing a traumatic event as a child. PTSD is clearly a disorder that is neither all biological nor all environmental. You must be exposed to an event that is overwhelming, but you probably must also have a brain that is vulnerable to extensive change as a result of such exposure. A better understanding of that vulnerability may lead to medications that protect against the possibility of PTSD later in life.

The Diagnosis

PTSD is much better documented and studied in adults than in children. For a diagnosis, a patient must have been exposed to a stressful event, after which impairing symptoms appear, including flashbacks about the event, emotional numbing, and a range of physical signs that can include sleep problems, survivor guilt, excessive reaction to unexpected events, and problems with memory or concentration.

Symptoms usually begin within three months of the trauma, and the course of the illness varies. Some people recover within six months, others have symptoms that last much longer. Not every traumatized person gets full-blown PTSD. It is diagnosed only if the symptoms last more than a month; in some cases, the condition is chronic.

These same symptoms apply to children who are victims of a single trauma, such as a serious car wreck or kidnapping. Younger children may not be able to express they are having a flashback; rather, they may exhibit an equivalent phenomenon called "traumatic play." For example, the well-known children's game ring-around-the-rosey is thought to be an example of traumatic play that originated during the Dark Ages in response to children observing the effects of the Black Plague. Alternately, a child who has been verbally or physically abused may repeatedly act out the abuse with dolls with an intensity suggesting that the child is trying to make the abuse more benign.

Diagnosing these symptoms in children exposed to more chronic forms of trauma, such as prolonged physical abuse or violent urban environments, can be more problematic. Many children do not have, or are at least unable to describe, clear flashbacks; instead, they may experience bouts of out-of-control behavior in reaction to minor frustrations. A better system of reliably identifying such symptoms, especially in young children, is needed.

Treatment

Children with PTSD can be helped by carefully targeted psychotherapy as well as with medication, if necessary.

Getting Help for Anxiety Disorders

In order to more effectively treat an anxiety disorder, a professional will want to get the most complete picture possible. **In making any diagnosis, a professional will:**

- Focus on the specific symptoms the child is suffering from
- Inquire about when the symptoms started and what their course has been (i.e. waxing and waning, constant, intermittent, steadily worsening)
- Ask what finally caused the family to seek treatment
- Try to put information in context. Is the family splitting up? Did a grandparent just die? Has the family moved recently? Is anything of note occurring in school?
- Perform an overall evaluation of the child's development

Mild anxiety problems can often be overcome at home, where parents acknowledge the child's distress and then create a comfortable situation in which the child can gradually deal with his or her fears. Should such efforts prove ineffective, you should consider seeking professional help.

Once you have consulted a professional, you might find they use similar strategies, generally called the behavioral approach or cognitive therapy. Depending on the child's age, the professional will try to identify the source of the anxiety by talking or playing with the child. Then, with the family's cooperation, they can make a plan for overcoming the fear. Part of that plan should include developing ways of deliberately dealing with fearful responses by both recognizing the symptoms and counteracting them. One way to counteract anxiety is to use relaxation techniques that slow breathing and help the mind focus on calming thoughts. For instance, a twelve-year-old who is fearful of spiders might first talk about spiders, then imagine what it would be like to be near a spider, and then think about having a spider on his arm or hand. The relaxation techniques help keep the fear at a tolerable level. Once imagining a spider is tolerable, the child repeats the exercise with a real spider, first in a cage at a distance and then gradually closer and closer until the spider actually is on the back of his hand.

Cognitive therapy also has a similar effect on more elaborate fears, such as speaking in public or dealing with obsessions and compulsions. The therapist and patient work together toward identifying a goal, create achievable steps toward that goal, and then take those steps together.

Medications

Medications can be helpful when anxiety becomes so overwhelming and debilitating that everyone feels helpless. Medications target the intense anxiety and the recurrent persistent thoughts, and, when effective, can produce rapid and sometimes total relief. However, they often only suppress the symptoms, so the patient must either continue taking medication indefinitely or risk a relapse. Also, simply preventing panic attacks or anxiety is often not enough to completely restore a person to normal life. Someone who has been housebound for several years is unlikely to suddenly go outside just because they are taking a medication to block panic attacks. That person must learn to do what he or she has been afraid of doing, and no medication can force that first step out the door.

Often, the medication recommended is an antidepressant. Families often find this confusing, because the child is anxious, not depressed. However, research has shown that most antidepressants also have powerful effects on the parts of the brain that deal with anxiety. The most common antidepressants used today are the selective serotonin reuptake inhibitors

(SSRIs). Low doses of these drugs have been shown to be helpful in treating anxiety disorders. Some antidepressants are sedating; others tend to be a bit stimulating. Such factors help dictate a choice, but the only sure way to know is to try it. Selecting the proper antidepressant can also involve considering likely side effects or other factors such as past family experience. If another family member with anxiety has done well on a particular antidepressant, evidence suggests it could work for the child too.

Occasionally, medications may be needed only for very brief interventions, like before a plane flight or medical procedure. In such cases, antianxiety agents can be a big help. However, some children experience an effect called disinhibition, which causes them to become disoriented and agitated. Because of such reactions, it is important to try medications out before the anxiety-causing event. Generally, it is useful to administer medications before the child starts getting anxious. It is much easier to calm a child at home and then go to the dentist's office than to have the child crying and screaming in fear at the office and then trying to give him medicine to help calm him there.

Sleeping Problems

There are many reasons to include sleeping problems in a chapter on anxiety. They frequently arise from anxiety disorders and, on those occasions when medication is used to treat sleeping problems, the types of medicines overlap with those used for treating anxiety. Like many forms of anxiety, sleep problems are usually approached nonpharmacologically at first. In my opinion, only serious sleeping issues that have resisted behavioral and structural interventions and are severely impairing the child's health or safety warrant medication as a treatment.

One of the "joys" of parenting is discovering how difficult it can be to get by on inadequate amounts of sleep. Our first son was awake every single night for the first eighteen months of his life, usually screaming inconsolably for at least one to two hours. Had you told me in advance that I could go that long without an uninterrupted night's sleep, I would have never believed you. Fortunately, most children accommodate to a night-and-day schedule a bit more rapidly than that, and doctors appropriately resist efforts to speed up the process with medication. (This was not, however, always so. In the early 1900s, many mothers helped their infants slumber with laudanum, the main active ingredient of which is opium.)

After infancy and between eighteen months and three years, a second wave of sleep difficulties can arise. The majority of these issues are simply manifestations of separation problems—the child doesn't want to be alone in a room with the lights out, and finds all sorts of way to delay that outcome (one more trip to the bathroom, another drink of water, fears about monsters under the bed, etc.). Most parents recognize what is happening and deal with it appropriately, setting firm but gentle limits while offering reassurance to their child.

Persistent patterns of such sleep resistance, especially if a child starts sleeping with his or her parents on a regular basis, warrant a consultation with a professional. Parents quickly come to recognize ways in which the rituals around bedtime increase everyone's anxiety rather than prepare the child for a restful night's sleep. Your pediatrician, child psychologist, or child and adolescent psychiatrist can help identify the source of the child's concerns and develop a plan for restoring a better bedtime routine. Behavioral changes, like these listed below, help the child transition to a quiet state that is conducive to sleep.

- **Choose quiet activities near bedtime, such as reading or listening to soothing music.** A vigorous game of tickle is not going to promote sleep readiness.
- **Let the child know well in advance**

that bedtime is coming. Abrupt transitions can be quite difficult for some children, so help them plan ahead.

- **Make sure that physical needs are met.** Children that are hungry, thirsty, need their diaper changed, or need to go to the bathroom are not apt to sleep.
- **Keep bedtime at a regular hour and stick to it.** Changing sleep time from night to night is confusing.
- **Create a reassuring sleep environment that reassures the child she is safe and loved.** Anxiety is a common cause of sleeping problems; help lower it as much as possible.
- **Once you've said good night, stay away!** Avoid the temptation of checking in to see how things are going. If the child comes out of his or her room, send him back firmly but gently.

Night Terrors

Night terrors, a frightening phenomenon that can occur with toddlers, is a sleep disorder related to a disruption of the normal physical paralysis that occurs during certain stages of sleep. A child with night terrors will begin to cry out and thrash about during the night. When parents respond to the child's distress, they may initially think he is awake because he may be sitting up with eyes open, but then typically find the child unresponsive to their voice or efforts to provide comfort. Usually, the child will awaken a few minutes later, frightened but unharmed. Rarely, night terrors can occur multiple times a night for many nights in a row, in which case formal assessment is appropriate and intervention with medications may be needed.

SLEEP HYGIENE

With older children and adolescents, "sleep hygiene" continues to be of major importance. Most studies of sleep needs suggest that the average child requires at least ten hours nightly, but the range is considerable. If you are the parent of a teenager, you already know from experience how few young people in this country come close to achieving that much sleep. Not only is it important to help ensure that your child gets adequate amounts of uninterrupted sleep, but also to encourage the same type of routine they had when they were younger. Even teenagers should be instructed to turn off the television or computer at least forty-five minutes before they want to be asleep. Washing up, brushing teeth, and climbing into bed to read a book or a magazine is a good way to become sleepy before turning out the light.

Persistent failure to get to sleep or stay asleep may be a symptom of a variety of disorders, including physical problems such as sleep apnea (obstruction of the airway during sleep) and psychiatric disorders such as depression and anxiety. It can also be a direct result of side effects from many of the medications used for treating psychiatric disorders. If sleep problems persist, consult with your child's pediatrician to address possible physical causes. If your child is on medication and the sleep problem began after it was started, ask the physician prescribing that medication if that could be the source of the problem.

The Bottom Line

The problem with anxiety is that it is so common we are tempted to assume it is normal. Parents generally assume that anxiety is something children will outgrow. That can certainly happen, but it is also something that can build upon itself. Why wait until your child has endured years of disabling fears that may grow into phobias or obsessions? Parents can be especially reluctant to seek help because they think they should be able to deal with a child who is easily overwhelmed or seems to fall apart over minor upsets or transitions. Similarly, a mother who, in desperation, has begun sleeping with her five-year-old every night to avoid endless trips back and forth between bedrooms may be convinced that telling a professional will only prove her incompetence. Be honest—professionals have heard and seen pretty much everything, and they want to help you as quickly as possible.

Chapter 7

Early Developmental Disorders

Early developmental disorders are specific conditions that interfere with your child's ability to reach certain expected milestones; they become apparent in the first few years of life. Just when most parents are reveling in the miracle of their new baby learning to walk and talk, parents of children with early developmental disorders are facing the slow realization that something is seriously wrong with their child. Why isn't she walking? Why does he no longer talk? Parents then begin to wonder if they are just imagining a problem or if there is something really wrong. But who do they ask? Where can they find help?

This chapter focuses on three disorders typically included under the general rubric of early developmental disorders: mental retardation, autism, and Asperger's disorder. While these are by no means the only causes of developmental delay, they are common diagnoses among the children I see for consultations about medication use. Furthermore, the medication issues are remarkably similar.

Early Signs

Developmental delay is not a diagnosis but a description of fact. A child with developmental delay fails to gain expected skills or competencies as compared to children who are roughly the same age. Some children show clear delays from early on; they learn to walk or talk late, and generally fail to meet other usual milestones. For others, early development seems, even in retrospect, nearly or completely normal, only to fall off markedly at eighteen to twenty-four months old, and sometimes even later. Even with clear delays, recognition of the severity of the problem is sometimes deferred for months or even years because parents hope the child will "snap out of it" or because pediatricians or other caregivers dismiss parental concerns.

These disorders are extremely challenging for families, and the advice in this chapter cannot possibly cover all the adjustments that may be necessary. The following descriptions are intended to help clarify why medications may be of value. For in-depth descriptions of the disorders and full explanations of all relevant treatments, refer to the resources in Appendix B (page 260). Because of the similarities of these disorders, their causes and treatments will be addressed collectively.

Mental Retardation

The term "mental retardation" brings fear to a parent's heart. The thought of raising a child with a lower-than-normal IQ is difficult for parents in our society. Whether you have dreams of your child attending Harvard or simply worry about your children not being able to live independently as adults, you already know our culture honors both beauty and intelligence. We all want our children to look like other children and have a normal IQ. While the most severe forms of mental retardation can be devastating, individuals who have less severe forms (which are far more common) may require some accommodations but can have relatively normal childhoods and become adults who lead independent, happy lives.

To be diagnosed as mentally retarded, a child must have a significantly low IQ (bottom 3 percent of all scores) that results in problems in adapting to everyday life. The most severe forms, with mental ages below age four, are typically caused by biological defects or injury; they account for less than 5 percent of all children with mental retardation. Remarkably, some disorders that cause mental retardation are completely preventable if detected early and treated appropriately. For example, a simple test is performed on every child born in the U.S. to detect a

DEGREES OF MENTAL RETARDATION

Borderline	IQ = 70 – 79
Mild	IQ = 50 – 69
Moderate	IQ = 35 – 49
Severe	IQ = 20 – 34
Profound	IQ < 20

genetic disorder called phenylketonuria, which can produce severe mental retardation unless dietary restrictions are instituted during the first few years of life. Causes of relatively milder forms of mental retardation may be genetic but can also be a result of environmental hardships, including a lack of exposure to stimuli that help promote learning.

Mental age is a process, not a steady state. In general, the lower the IQ, the longer it takes to reach any given developmental level and the sooner intellectual development stops. A child with an IQ of 100 should have a mental age of two years at age two, five years at age five, etc. New skills continue to emerge until about age sixteen. For someone with an IQ of 50, it takes roughly twice as long to reach any given developmental level as for someone with an IQ of 100. Furthermore, cognitive development typically hits its ceiling at a younger age, perhaps twelve or fourteen

years. For all of us, even after cognitive development has peaked, we still can learn new areas of expertise, increase our vocabulary, etc., but our basic brainpower is fixed.

There is really no distinct line between being mentally retarded and normal. Furthermore, results on a specific IQ tests may pick up only a fraction of a person's functional strengths and weaknesses. For example, if IQ tests were based on artistic ability rather than verbal skill, my current mental age would be, at best, about six or seven. Parents and professionals in the 1950s and 60s fought hard to prove that the majority of children with mental retardation can lead quite productive and satisfying lives, given appropriate support and opportunities.

Mental retardation is largely untreatable, at least in the sense of "curing" it with medication. However, it is also frequently accompanied by ADHD, anxiety disorders,

DEVELOPMENT, IQ SCORES, AND BRAIN FUNCTION

All of us know that children change—over time, they grow larger, they learn to talk, and they acquire various skills. Despite lots of individual differences, these changes happen in relatively predictable ways. A child who walks at ten months is "early," while a child who walks at seventeen months is "late;" from a medical perspective, however, a child who walks at any time within this range is considered "normal."

Development is definitely not a smooth ramp along which all children progress evenly. Rather, it is more like a series of steps, with each subsequent developmental achievement being based on previous ones. These achievements are typically the result of complex interactions between brain development and environmental opportunities.

The process of learning to walk is a good example of the importance of brain function. No matter how hard you try, you can't teach a normal six-month-old to walk; certain changes in the spinal neurons must occur first. On average, children who crawl early also walk early, but there is no way to know when a child will start walking based on when he learned to crawl. And some children never crawl—they just suddenly begin walking.

In the early part of the twentieth century, researchers measured the abilities of thousands of individuals at different ages and constructed the concept of mental age. For example, an average ten-year-old who can do pretty much everything any other child his age can do has a mental age (MA) of 10 and a real or chronological age (CA) of 10. His IQ, or intelligence quotient, is 100, as determined by this formula:

$$MA/CA \times 100 = IQ*$$
$$10/10 \times 100 = 100$$

Suppose the child can do almost everything the average fourteen-year-old can do:

$$14/10 \times 100 = 140$$

That makes the child highly intelligent.

Most of us have an IQ somewhere in the normal range, between 80 and 120. But, just as some children are brighter than average, others are less bright. Suppose another ten-year-old turns out to have a mental age of six years, four years, or even lower. These are the children who receive a diagnosis of mental retardation (see table on degrees of mental retardation).

---

*This equation works well only up to about age 10; in practice, psychologists use tables to determine IQ, but the concept is the same.

depression, and obsessive-compulsive disorder, all of which can be treated if they are recognized.

Autism

Children with autism are characteristically disinterested in and unresponsive to social interactions and have delays in communication that range from no functional speech to odd and idiosyncratic language. Many also have strikingly odd behaviors, including an all-consuming interest in aspects of an object such as its feel, form, or color. They might also engage in repetitive behaviors, such as spinning or twirling in circles, banging their head, or flapping their hands. Some have an overwhelming need for sameness in environment or routines. Older children with normal or superior intelligence may manifest these oddities in strange interests, such as memorizing the height of every professional basketball player or the birthdates of famous people.

Autism was first documented in the mid-1940s by Leo Kanner, a pioneering child psychiatrist. Since then, it has gone from being thought of as a rare disorder to one that is diagnosed with far greater frequency. Until the late 1980s, autism and mental retardation where thought to be strongly linked. It is still true that nearly all children diagnosed with autism also have some degree of mental retardation; however, research has shown that similar oddities in social interaction, language, and behavior can be present in individuals with normal or even superior intelligence.

These similarities led clinicians to start looking at the symptoms of autism as a function of the child's mental age. Just as a two-year-old does not have the same types of social relationships as a six- or ten-year-old, expectations should be adjusted based on a patient's mental age. A four-year-old autistic child who has a mental age of two may be only beginning to acquire useful language and have fairly rudimentary obsessive behavior, such as lining up blocks. At age ten and with a mental age of five, that same child may have much richer language with continued oddities such as echolalia (constant repetition of words or phrases), poor or no use of pronouns such as "I" and "you," and little to no ability to engage in a conversation. The habit of lining up blocks may have progressed to something a bit more sophisticated but still similar; for example, insisting on keeping a group of favorite videotapes in precise order. The disorder is essentially unchanged, but the mental age has altered how it looks.

What Is It?

No test exists for autism. In the U.S.,

autism is typically diagnosed when a child is between the ages of two and four. It can be hard to diagnose because the disorder manifests itself in many ways. Retrospective studies suggest that many children with autism have odd behaviors possibly from birth, but about one-third seem to develop normally until about eighteen to twenty-four months of age. At that point, cognitive development stops or regresses, with loss of language, social isolation, and the emergence of odd behaviors. An accurate diagnosis requires considerable expertise, as none of the symptoms used to make the diagnosis are specific for autism and most are highly dependent on mental age.

The most noticeable characteristics of autism include:

- **Social isolation.** Autistic children are generally withdrawn and aloof and fail to respond to other people. These children are frequently described as "being in their own world." They have a lack of social awareness or interest in others and may avoid eye contact. To the autistic, people and objects are interchangeable. There may be a lack of interacting with the mother from infancy, even when breastfeeding. These children tend not to approach parents for comfort or engage in any of the normal patterns of parent-child interaction.

- **Severe language delays.** Some children may acquire limited language until they are eighteen to twenty-four months old, and then lose some or all of what they have acquired. Others simply have few language skills. For this reason, many parents visit the pediatrician, worried that the child has a hearing problem. Those children who do speak may exhibit unusual speech patterns, such as speaking in a monotone, in rhyme, or in repetitive phrases they have heard. Around 40 to 60 percent of children with autism never develop meaningful speech, or they have a very limited vocabulary. The ability to understand speech (called receptive language) may also be impaired, but usually less so than expressive language.

- **Odd behaviors.** Many, but not all, children with autism exhibit behaviors that are notably unusual or odd. For example, they may persist in endless rocking, flapping, spinning, hair twirling, head banging, or self-biting. Some adopt a tiptoe walk that can cause problems with the Achilles tendon that eventually necessitates surgery. Other odd behaviors include obsessive manipulations of objects, like lining blocks up in a very specific way or trying to spin any object they can reach. Some children also show a rigid need for routine and sameness;

for example, they may explode into anger if a parent tries to take a different route home from school or if an object in their bedroom is displaced. The cause or purpose of these odd behaviors is not well understood, but they are so striking that they quickly raise the question of autism.

While these characteristics are the primary ones used to diagnose autism, many autistic children also have abnormal responses to sensory stimuli. Some may exhibit heightened sensitivity to sound, covering their ears to mute certain noises; others are so unresponsive to noises that parents worry they are deaf. Loud and close noises may produce no reaction, while minor noises at a different pitch may induce tantrums, even when they occur at a distance. Some children will eat only certain kinds of food based on texture, chewiness, or color. Some cannot tolerate certain kinds of fabrics or tags on clothing.

Severity and Outcome of Autism

There is no universal measurement of the severity of autism, although one often hears about mild, moderate, or severe forms of the disorder. Usually, such terms refer to the degree of concurrent mental retardation; that is, mild cases include only autism with normal or superior intellectual functioning, while severe cases have mental ages far below actual age. Alternatively, autism is sometimes ranked on the basis of the perceived intensity of its symptoms. Thus a child with severe autism might be one who has absolutely no interest in or ability to make use of social interactions with other people, while a child with mild autism might have adequate relations with supportive adults but be unable to navigate the complexity of peer interactions.

Some autistic children are very bright and do well in school, though they may have difficulty with social adjustment and some types of reasoning. The majority, however, have some level of accompanying mental retardation. In my experience, autism seems to affect day-to-day functional ability by roughly one level in the ranking of severity of mental retardation (see table on degrees of mental retardation). Thus, an autistic individual who has an IQ of 100 tends to function in many ways like someone with mild mental retardation.

The ability to communicate is an especially important factor for diagnosing autism. Children with autism typically have marked delays both in receptive speech and expressive speech; that is, what they absorb and how they communicate. Some autistic children will finally begin to develop speech at three or four years of age; however, if a child still has no speech by age six, it is unlikely that he ever will.

Many children with autism will do all they can to avoid using language. I often use the phrase "lack of communicative drive" to describe this reluctance to speak. It is one of the characteristics that distinguishes a child with autism from one with speech delays. Children with speech delays almost always grasp the importance of communicating long before they have much of an ability to do so, and will use whatever few words and gestures they can to convey their wishes. In sharp contrast, those with autism typically first try to meet their own needs; next, they may use nonverbal efforts, such as hand pulling or pushing, to get someone else to meet a need they cannot satisfy themselves; and only as a reluctant last choice will they turn to speech.

Autistic Savants

The abilities of autistic patients I've seen run the gamut. I've met with families whose children were totally unresponsive and uncommunicative; others have been totally out of control. Some can be remarkably high-functioning and yet still have tremendous problems. For example, I once met with a sixteen-year-old whose family brought him to see me. When the appointment time arrived, my office door suddenly opened and an intense young man barged into my office, sat down in the chair across from me, and—without introducing himself or indicating that he knew who I was—blurted out, "I know the winner of every World Series since 1903. Pick a year." Indeed, he knew every World Series winner, and many other details of professional baseball. What he did not know, despite an IQ of 135, was how to engage in a meaningful conversation with another human being. He'd gone his whole life without a proper diagnosis because, at the time, the manifestations of the disorder in people of such high intelligence were only beginning to be understood.

One rare and poorly understood phenomenon sometimes seen in individuals with autism is the presence of splinter skills. Adolescents or adults with these skills generally seem to function at a mental age of two or three and yet display exceptional abilities as artists, sculptors, or musicians. Also impressive are individuals who are not so severely delayed but have other exceptional skills, such as "calendar ability." They can tell you on what day of the week any specified date will occur—or, more rarely, remember with remarkable clarity not only the day of the week of any past date but also exactly where they were and what the weather was like.

Other individuals, because of their intense interests, can recite with exactitude information that most of us can't keep in our heads. For example, a young man in the San Francisco area is a regular on one of the early morning talk shows. When given two destinations anywhere in the Bay Area, he can rapidly describe exactly what trains, buses, ferries, or other means of public transportation are needed to get from one place to the other—including time schedules. Individuals with such abilities sometimes are called "autistic savants," and parents with such children are understandably both proud of and baffled by the dichotomy. In some arenas, these children can perform brilliantly, yet they suffer overwhelming delays in the areas of basic functioning we normally deem essential.

Rising Numbers

Everyone agrees that the number of children now being diagnosed with autism and Asperger's disorder, a closely related disorder, has risen dramatically over the past fifteen years. Some assert that as many as one in every one hundred children may now have so-called "autism spectrum disorders;" that is, not only autism itself but other, milder problems with socialization and odd behaviors. Indeed, this is a significant increase from the estimates of one in five or ten thousand cited in the mid-1980s.

Theories about this dramatic change are abundant and unproven. For example, some argue that the rise is a direct result from changes in how the disorder is diagnosed. Others worry that a change in the environment, ranging from increased use of artificial additives in food to widespread use of childhood immunizations, is responsible. Those who might wonder why there is no answer yet should consider how the world has changed in the past fifteen to twenty years. Potentially, any of those changes might have a role, alone or in combination with other factors.

To date, research on immunizations, perhaps the scariest theory for parents, has resoundingly failed to show any association between autism and either the vaccinations themselves or ingredients in those vaccinations. Whatever the reasons for change, most reputable textbooks on autism now cite an occurrence of about one in every thousand births.

Asperger's Disorder

Asperger's disorder is similar to autism, but most children with Asperger's have normal intelligence. By definition, they must have developed normal language skills by age three, although almost all exhibit odd speech patterns. Some speak in a monotone; others have a musical quality to their speech. Those with Asperger's are often loners and invariably have trouble with social interactions, especially with

THE DEBATE OVER NORMAL

Part of the debate about the prevalence of autism, and particularly of Asperger's disorder, arises from uncertainties about when social isolation is normal. Is every eight-year-old who has trouble making friends and prefers to spend all her time obsessing over the latest video game on the autism spectrum? What about eccentric figures such as Bill Gates or Albert Einstein? If we choose to broaden the diagnosis to include such individuals, does that support or weaken the theory that we are in the midst of an epidemic?

Concerns about the line between normal and abnormal arise from both sides of the divide. What is the value of labeling an individual who happens to prefer solitary time over social mingling and has an intense interest in a singular topic? If he or she does not perceive a problem, why should we insist that there is one? Even if there is some evidence of a problem, how does it help to say, in essence, "Of course you feel this way—you have Asperger's disorder"? In this instance, the label is of little consolation to either child or parent. Similarly, is the importance of accurately labeling children and adolescents who do have a serious developmental disorder devalued if those same labels are applied to people who function well?

peers. They typically show little empathy, although this may have more to do with a failure to notice or appreciate distress in others rather than an inability to feel distress from emotional situations. Although not used as a criterion for the diagnosis, children with Asperger's often have poor motor skills, making them appear clumsy and unable to use their hands for more precise activities, especially when young. Like autistic children, these children may also have odd behaviors. They are very likely to focus totally on a particular issue, usually one with a heavy focus on facts, figures, or other parts of the environment, as opposed to people.

Asperger's disorder was identified as a distinct syndrome only about fifteen years ago, and there still is considerable debate as to its relationship to autism. Some believe that it is a distinct syndrome; others argue that it is just autism with higher intelligence and without the speech delays. Typically, neither language nor other aspects of early development are delayed in children with Asperger's, so diagnosis often doesn't occur until a child is at least four or five, and sometimes considerably later. In fact, parents and other adults are often enchanted with these children because of their early, obsessive interest in letters, numbers, and order.

A few years ago, I was asked to consult on an eight-year-old boy, Pete, because his parents were concerned he might have ADHD. It turned out that Pete had Asperger's disorder. With considerable parental support, he had done well enough in a private school that he made it to third grade without a teacher requesting he see a mental health specialist. However, a review of his history made it clear that he was very socially isolated, showed no interest in birthdays or other holidays, and he generally avoided extreme expressions of emotion of any kind. His peers had shunned him, calling him "weird," which was fine with him, because he much preferred playing by himself.

Another remarkable child who came to my office brought with him a chain full of car keys that he had been collecting for years. The collection must have weighed two pounds, and he knew exactly what type of car each key fit. This nine-year-old's favorite topic of conversation, of course, was cars; as soon as you told him what brand of car you drove, he could begin reciting all its features, such as sound systems, moonroof, leather interior, etc. For a twelve-year-old boy I saw recently, it was elevators and fans. Breathlessly, he started telling me about Web sites he had found where he could memorize the exact dimensions of various elevators or the length of blades for different models of ceiling fans.

The key point is not the obsessive fascination these children exhibit, for many young boys and girls go through phases of being intensely interested in a topic or activity. Rather, it is the mechanical or statistical aspect of the subjects that seem to attract individuals with Asperger's, as well as the way it develops in complete social isolation. It stands in sharp contrast to a child who is "obsessed" with the latest collector cards or video games, which almost invariably have a significant interactive component with peers, or even adults, that helps to sustain the interest.

Because of their intelligence level and ability to communicate, the outlook for children with Asperger's disorder is generally more optimistic than for those who are autistic. However, that does not mean the disorder is a minor one; many children with Asperger's are so inflexible and unable to engage in acceptable social interactions that normal interactions can be difficult, if not impossible.

In DSM-IV, both autism and Asperger's disorder fall into a broader category called pervasive developmental disorder (PDD). Individuals who meet some of the criteria for either autism or Asperger's, but not enough to qualify for a diagnosis, may receive a diagnosis of "pervasive developmental disorder, not otherwise specified," or PDDNOS. The term "PDD" is commonly used to refer either to a patient with PDDNOS or to the entire category of individuals with any of these disorders. More recently, the term "autism spectrum disorders" has emerged as an alternative that encompasses the entire population with autism, Asperger's, and PDDNOS.

Causes of Early Developmental Delays

There is no single cause for the disorders that produce early developmental delays. Genetics can play a role, especially for certain inheritable forms of mental retardation and some types of autism. Prenatal testing can detect an array of common causes for mental retardation, but not for autism or Asperger's. With rare exceptions, early developmental disorders are much more common in boys; the male-to-female ratio for autism is about four boys to every girl.

Mental retardation alone can have literally hundreds of causes. These include inherited and random genetic variants that produce disruptions in normal brain development: exposure to drugs, tobacco, and alcohol during pregnancy; trauma resulting from difficult birth; early exposure to toxins, viruses, and other agents that directly damage the brain; and physical injuries resulting directly from accidental or

deliberate trauma to the head or indirectly through prolonged lack of oxygen. In addition, persistent deprivation either of vital nutrients or environmental stimulation can lead to cognitive delays. Thus, many children rescued from orphanages in eastern European countries after the fall of communism there showed significant mental retardation. This was probably due to a combination of extremely poor nutrition and severe neglect—most of these children were in overcrowded facilities where there was little food and many spent days unattended in cribs. Sometimes the effects of neglect and deprivation are reversible with improved nutrition and environment, but not always. Typically, however, the most severe levels of mental retardation are genetic, metabolic, or traumatic in origin.

Professionals in the field now largely agree that autism and Asperger's disorder are a result of brain dysfunction, and early theories that it arose from a severe problem of attachment caused by cold, unfeeling mothers have been thoroughly discredited. Despite a range of factors, there is still no convincing theory of what causes autism or Asperger's. There is evidence of a genetic influence in some families, and exposure to certain viruses early in fetal development can markedly increase the risk of developing autism accompanied by severe mental retardation.

However, the parts of the brain involved or what kind of dysfunction they might create remains a mystery, and the tools needed to study this problem are still being developed.

One of the early efforts to understand the causes of autism involved studies of neurotransmitters, the chemicals in the brain that convey information from one nerve cell to another. In the mid-1960s, it was discovered that levels of the neurotransmitter serotonin were abnormally high in one-third of autistic individuals. However, extensive efforts to show a connection to autism or to treat it by correcting this elevation with drugs have failed. Studies of other neurotransmitters known to be important to brain function have been equally unrewarding.

Another line of persistent inquiry has been the theory that autism is a result of a toxin that inflicts nonspecific, but severe, damage to the brain. A recent example is the hypothesis that autism is a result of the mercury preservative used in childhood vaccines. Even though a study completed by the Institute of Medicine in May 2004 showed no link between autism and vaccines, many parents still fear they have done something to cause their child's autism. Similar hypotheses propose there is a flaw in the intestines that allows absorption of various toxins which then damage the brain. Again, evidence supporting such explanations remains scientifically unconvincing.

Technological advances now are enabling researchers to undertake brain-imaging studies to further investigate the underlying cause of these disorders. Although autism is generally not diagnosed until a child is about eighteen months old, scientists are finding that there are subtle brain abnormalities from birth. For example, multiple regions of the brain, including the size of the ventricles (fluid cavities) appear different in these children. The root of the problem, however, might be in the "wiring" of the brain—parts of the brain develop too many connections, and other parts too few. In many cases, the various parts of the brain work well independently, but they just can't connect to each other. Later on, the affected areas show signs of inflammation, and this condition seems to be permanent. One researcher compares this theory to circuit boards that may be intact, but have mixed-up connecting cables.

Although highly intriguing, these types of studies only reflect trends. Lots of children with autism do not have the abnormalities described. Furthermore, none of these discoveries have led to any immediate treatments or suggested ways of preventing the occurrence of autism or Asperger's disorder.

IF YOU THINK YOUR CHILD ISN'T PROGRESSING NORMALLY

Many parents worry if their child doesn't walk precisely at twelve months or talk at fifteen months. Before becoming unduly alarmed, take a step back and think about your child's development, and consider the following:

• Many excellent books give good guidelines about what to expect at each stage of development. However, they all emphasize the importance of individual variability in the timing of new skills.

• Change and acquisition of new skills are integral to early development. If an infant or toddler stops gaining new abilities for more than a month or two, or actually loses an emerging skill, it is not unreasonable to seek out professional advice. An eighteen-month-old who is pointing and has good command of a dozen or so words does not typically withdraw and stop talking. (This is in sharp contrast to the ten- or twelve-month-old who once said something the parents were convinced was "hamburger" but who then returned to babbling and saying "mama" and "dada.")

• If you are convinced that your child is truly developing at a very different pace from his or her peers, make a special appointment to see the pediatrician.

• Look for converging opinions from people with experience. First-time parents tend to worry excessively, but they also may convince themselves their child is doing fine because they lack experience. I was involved in a study many years ago that found that, on average, first-time parents waited about twelve months longer before seeking help with a child ultimately diagnosed with autism than parents with more than one child. If grandparents, friends with children, or preschool teachers are saying something is wrong, ask them to explain what they are seeing and how that differs from other children the same age.

• Do not let physicians and other diagnosticians browbeat you into silence. If you are worried about a specific behavior or lack of emerging skill and the doctor tells you to stop worrying, ask why she is not concerned and when you do need to worry. If you remain unconvinced, explore at least one other option for further assessment.

• If your child is ultimately diagnosed with a delay but you hesitated to see someone because you were unsure, don't panic. Essentially, all of the disorders that cause early developmental delays are slowly progressive problems for which few, if any, specific treatments exist. Some are impossible to diagnose until the child has reached a mental age where certain key signs or symptoms emerge.

Getting a Proper Diagnosis

Most pediatricians and family health care practitioners are not experts in diagnosing the details of specific developmental problems beyond establishing known causes of mental retardation and ruling out possible vision and hearing problems. Typically, they refer families to those who can provide more information, like child and adolescent psychiatrists or child psychologists. These professionals administer the type of developmental testing that helps generate accurate diagnoses and forms the basis for planning interventions.

As mentioned earlier, mental retardation has a variety of identifiable causes for which precise laboratory tests exist. Such examinations are almost always recommended as part of a screening for severe developmental delays. There are no biological or genetic tests yet for either autism or Asperger's disorder, although some screening questionnaires are used to assess the presence or absence of concerning or symptomatic behaviors. In addition, various methods exist for pinpointing where a child is functioning along developmental lines such as physical abilities, language, and social skills. These methods can provide more precise information as to where a child may be having difficulties, as well as monitoring the child's progress.

Treatment Possibilities

Treatment of mental retardation is largely preventative, as previously discussed, and facilitative (helping the individual to maximize potential and independence). Until the 1950s, children with any significant degree of mental retardation were removed from the home, usually at an early age, and placed in state institutions. Many of these institutions were poorly funded and dedicated mainly to warehousing individuals for their whole lives. This picture began changing dramatically during the 1950s and '60s, and now these large-scale state institutions have virtually vanished.

Now, most American children with mental retardation stay with their families, who utilize a range of state-funded programs to help them maximize their child's potential. Programs for children under age three are typically provided by independent organizations using state and federal funding to provide early interventions, including helping children learn at developmentally appropriate rates and helping parents better understand their child's needs. The school system becomes heavily involved in educating children over age three, and that responsibility continues to some extent until the child's twenty-third birthday (in most states). Programs exist in many communities to provide small-group housing for teenagers who are seeking greater independence or cannot stay with their families because of behavioral problems. Again, in most states, these programs are supported with public funds.

Emotional and behavioral disorders may also be associated with mental retardation, and they may interfere with the child's function and development. As they get older, these children may grow aware of their differences and become frustrated, withdrawn, or anxious. Dealing with these problems on an issue-by-issue basis may make life easier, and your pediatrician may recommend visits to other specialists to help with hearing, speech, sight, or physical or emotional difficulties.

Autism and Asperger's

Although not everyone agrees, I believe that autism and Asperger's disorder are problems for which we do not have any true cures. It is a common and extremely frustrating experience to speak with parents who insist that their child must have autism, rather than mental retardation, because they believe the former is more treatable than the latter. Unfortunately, changing the label does nothing about the actual problem. I have higher hopes for a child with mental retardation than for a similar child with autism, in terms of

continued development and long-term results. Children with Asperger's usually have a better prognosis than those with the other two diagnoses because of a higher level of intellectual functioning, but they too can have persistent problems that are difficult or impossible to overcome.

Since autism is typically diagnosed in young children, initial interventions focus on behavioral control and language development. The degree of coexisting mental retardation plays a crucial role in program planning because interventions need to be tailored to the child's mental age. The biggest differences between programs for children with mental retardation and those with autism reflect the central problem with autism—lack of social interest. Autistic children tend not to be motivated to please adults; they are much more likely to try to avoid them and their peers as well. Programs for these children focus on individual work using motivating rewards, such as food. Also, many autistic children do better processing information through their eyes than through their ears, so visual cues can be helpful. These children typically do much better when they can follow familiar routines and repeat activities over and over.

Unlike mentally retarded children, children with Asperger's disorder are typically diagnosed later and usually have problems not directly related to their mental abilities. In part because this disorder was recognized only recently, there is much less uniformity among programs for these children. They too can have problems in school but not usually because of the learning skills. Instead, in late elementary school and beyond, they typically have problems with both peer skills and with comprehension and creativity demands. Problems like these can include reading well above age level but being unable to comprehend how to write even a brief essay on a chosen topic. The child might also refuse to study anything not directly related to his specific interest or become overwhelmed when a teacher asks him to present "everything you can learn about your state," and he cannot distinguish the important information from the unimportant in the materials he has read.

Socially, many of these children do relatively well with adults, who admire their intellect and tolerate their odd interests, but extremely poorly with same-age peers, who just think they are weird. Some efforts exist to improve social interactions by direct teaching of social skills in small groups, and these can be of some help.

Behavior Modification

One technique that has proven to be of

APPLIED BEHAVIOR ANALYSIS

One of the more dramatic applications of behavioral modification to an early developmental disorder was pioneered in the early 1980s by a UCLA researcher named Dr. O. Ivar Lovaas. Now called discrete trial learning and applied behavior analysis (ABA) training, this method theorized that intensive behavior intervention could "break through the wall" that autistic children put around themselves, resulting in improvements in the disorder. Dr. Lovaas devised an intervention that focused initially on compliance (getting the child to do what adult trainers asked), using a combination of positive rewards for correct responses and physical coercion, if needed. Usually the initial rewards were quite basic—typically foods the child liked. The reward was then accompanied by praise that could itself be used as a reward later on. Lovaas showed that after an initial, often intense resistance, many of the children he studied became far more compliant and were able to learn new skills in language and social interactions using the same techniques. In his first published study, he described an intervention that lasted forty hours a week for two years. He showed improvement in some, but not all children studied, in cognitive skills such as language and academic subjects, and in social interactions as well. After treatment some of his subjects no longer even met the criteria for autism.

considerable value for all early developmental disorders is behavioral modification. In fact, this approach has also been useful in many other aspects of treating mental disorders and even assisting parents with children who don't have a psychiatric disorder. The principles are relatively easy to explain; but, as is often the case with simple ideas, successful application can require some level of expertise and persistence. Over the past several decades, clinicians and researchers have worked out these **key rules for successful behavioral modification:**

- Pick a specific behavior to change.
- Choose motivating reinforcements.
- Use positive reinforcement
  when possible.
- Be consistent.
- Be persistent.
- Maintain the program long enough to
  create permanent change.

Many parents are intimidated by such programs, but the evidence of success can be a powerful motivating factor for behavioral change. Most programs for children with developmental delays have behaviorists available to help parents master the principles and apply them to their specific concern.

It is not unreasonable to ask why every child with autism is not receiving this type of intervention. The answer is complex. First, it is unclear whether every child with autism either needs this level of intervention or would benefit from it. It seems most effective at breaking down the social barrier that the most severely autistic children have, where the child shows no interest at all in people. For children with less severe isolation issues, such interventions may have little benefit. Second, it may help with problems of compliance as do other, less intense applications of behavioral interventions, but there is no evidence that it can affect cognitive ability. In other words, it cannot increase the mental age of a child with mental retardation. Third, like any powerful intervention, it can have negative as well as positive effects, especially if used to force children to perform feats they simply cannot do. Imagine, for example, being pushed eight hours a day, forty hours a week, month after month, to learn to jump fifty feet in a single bound—on one leg—with no recourse. Last, this type of intervention is extremely expensive. Few families can afford the private sessions, most insurance policies will not cover it, and school and other public agencies lack funding to offer it to every child. Efforts are underway to see what level of intensity of intervention is actually needed as well as how best to identify those who can truly benefit from it.

Medications and Similar Interventions

. . . .

Although there are no medications that can cure any of the common causes of early developmental delay, there are a number of behaviors common to these disorders which medications can treat:

- **For unmanageable agitation, aggression, or rage**—antipsychotics, mood stabilizers, beta-blockers, antidepressants
- **For self-mutilation and head banging**—antipsychotics, low-dose SSRIs, naltrexone
- **For severe impulsivity**—stimulants, antipsychotics, lithium, antidepressants
- **For obsessive-compulsive behaviors**—SSRIs, possibly atypical antipsychotics
- **For perseverative behaviors such as rocking or twirling or playing with an object for hours**—antipsychotics, antidepressants
- **For labile mood with temper outbursts**—antipsychotics, antidepressants

Whenever feasible, the medicating doctor should attempt to find one medication that can address multiple problems. With patients who have little to no language, you and your doctor may have to use a trial-and-error method of finding the correct medication, which can be more taxing than with other types of disorders. Multiple medications are another factor that can complicate the problem; if your child is taking one type of medication and another is added, it becomes increasingly difficult to evaluate the drug's efficacy, since drug interactions are sometimes difficult to identify.

Classes of Medications for Autism

Stimulants are generally not effective for autism because problems with attention and impulsivity may simply reflect mental age. However, a prescribing doctor may use them for treatment in a very limited circumstance. Unfortunately, there may be an increase in agitated motor activity lasting six to eight hours. Antidepressants can be quite effective in treating obsessive behaviors, which are common in both autism and Asperger's disorder. Studies have shown that some SSRIs, such as fluoxetine and sertraline, can cause restlessness, so they should not be a first choice for these children. While many parents express concern about using antidepressants because of reports regarding suicidal tendencies, this issue has not been studied among the autistic.

Antipsychotic medications for calming purposes have been used effectively for several decades with autistic patients. Still, parents face potentially difficult de-

WHEN TO MEDICATE

Medication should be considered when it can remove or lessen the underlying cause of an undesirable behavior or when a child's behavior is clearly dangerous to self or others or impairs learning. It should also be considered if other nondrug approaches have been unsuccessful. For instance, if a child is having explosive tantrums because she cannot satisfy her obsessive urges, reduction of those urges may calm the tantrums. A child who won't stop hitting his head against the wall and who has not responded to behavioral approaches may also benefit from medication. Unfortunately, I have found that it is possible to identify an underlying cause only about a quarter of the time. In the remaining cases, the goal becomes calming the child so he is less likely to engage in self-injury, tantrums, or other disruptive behaviors. The goal is not to "dull out" the child, and I emphasize to parents that such "dulling out" is an unacceptable side effect for which we need to watch carefully. If behavior suppression is absolutely necessary, then adequate control is preferable to optimal control.

Especially with new-onset behaviors, such as head banging, it is important to ask the pediatrician to conduct a full examination to rule out any physical causes. Has the child suffered a recent injury, or is there any possibility of infection in the ears, sinuses, or bladder? If so, they should be treated appropriately. Seizures are also a possibility, and they, too, have specific treatments. (One-third of children with autism have seizures by their mid-teens.)

When considering the possibility of medication, keep these questions in mind:

- What age is the child?

- Is the behavior that you are considering medication for mild or severe? If the behavior is only a little annoying and doesn't impair function, it may be worth holding out.

- Is the behavior new or chronic? If new, what has changed? If chronic, why should it be addressed now?

- Where does the behavior occur? If only in one setting, why there?

- Are there clear causes for the behavior, such as transitions, intentional or accidental interruptions of obsessive activities, loud or startling noises, or simple demands?

Parents must be on the alert for side effects, especially with autistic children whose communication skills are poor. Parents also need to watch for adverse side effects, which may bring out other undesirable behaviors, or may become more bothersome as other medications are added.

cisions. Older antipsychotics such as haloperidol (Haldol) produce a range of acute side effects, such as muscle spasms, and also carry the long-term risk of producing a movement disorder called tardive dyskinesia (TD).

Mood stabilizers are not generally used with autistic children. Blood levels need to be carefully monitored, which makes it a more complex drug to use and track.

Using Medications to Treat Common Problems

Some 25 to 70 percent of patients with major developmental disorders may need and can benefit from psychoactive medications, depending on the diagnosis, age, and behavioral problems of the patient. Once a medication has been started, it almost always needs to be used chronically to maintain the benefit. As mentioned earlier, the great majority of medications used for treating children and adolescents who have developmental delays do not have FDA endorsement for the specific usages discussed here. At present, interest in medications for the autistic is outstripping the pace at which they can be fully researched, and this can compromise safety.

DEALING WITH DEVELOPMENTAL DELAYS

One reason I will occasionally agree to prescribe medication for a young child with developmental delays is persistent sleep problems that can put the entire family at risk. For example, one four-and-a-half-year-old patient with moderate mental retardation had problems sleeping, and usually got no more than a few hours at a time. His parents finally came to me after he had gotten up in the middle of the night and gone into the kitchen. He had dumped every available bottle, carton, and box onto the floor, covering himself and everything else in syrup, flour, and a variety of other foodstuffs. His parents took this destruction fairly well but were aware that next time he might get interested in the stove or find a sharp knife. He shared a room with his younger brother, and they were worried about that son's safety, too. Furthermore, they lived in an apartment and worried that if they tried to lock him into room at night, he would make so much noise they might lose the apartment. They were content with his program otherwise and just wanted him to be able to sleep through the night. After making sure they had exhausted all other reasonable options, I agreed to talk with them about a medication trial. We discussed several possibilities but finally agreed on a trial of trazodone, an antidepressant that also acts as a sedative. The medication helped him go to sleep more easily and stay asleep until morning. To everyone's surprise, he also seemed to benefit during the day, showing less irritability and at least a modest improvement in concentration at school.

I seldom agree to use medications for children under age six, although I will admit that age is arbitrary. Since considerable development of brain neurotransmitters continues through the first few years of life and medication use in older children is more extensive than in younger ones, it seems wise to avoid potential problems wherever possible.

After age six or seven, the criteria for appropriate medications begins to change. Children are bigger, so behaviors that might have been unpleasant earlier can escalate to dangerous actions like aggressive biting, hitting, or impulsive actions, such as darting out into streets. In addition, behavioral interventions have usually been in place for some time, so parents and other professionals have had a chance to evaluate their success. Also, demands on the child continue to rise at home and at school, which may highlight difficulties with impulsivity and inattention or cause problems such as anxiety or depression.

For a new patient and family, I always begin with a medication consultation. This includes an exploration of the specific behavior or behaviors causing the problem as well as the details about when these behaviors started, when they occur, and when they stop. I am always suspicious of new behaviors, because they typically result from a change that needs to be identified and corrected, if

possible. For example, at age eight, Jake, who is autistic, mildly mentally retarded, and has no language, suddenly began repeatedly hitting his face hard right under his eye with the palms of both hands. Although self-injurious behaviors are quite common in children like Jake, this was unusual because of its abrupt onset. I suggested a medical examination—not easy with this child—and the pediatrician discovered that Jake had a severe sinus infection right at the spot where he was hitting himself. For him, the proper prescription was an antibiotic.

Jill's family, on the other hand, reluctantly came to see me because her school had sent them. Jill, age twelve, had autism with normal intelligence but limited language skills and was in a program to integrate her into a regular classroom, for at least part of the day. However, a few weeks after this program started, she would inexplicably fly into a rage after entering the regular class, attacking whichever child was nearest to her. The school was highly distressed and insisted the family find a medication to stop this from happening. Jill's parents were quite clear that this type of behavior was most unusual for her and that they never had such problems at home.

Further discussion revealed that the school's response to Jill's attacks was to scold her and then punish her by sending her back to her resource classroom, which she loved. In short, they had created the perfect behavioral program for teaching her to attack other children: They put her into an unpleasant program and reward her aggressions promptly by returning her to a comfortable, familiar environment. We spoke with the school about stopping the mainstreaming effort for a while, which quelled her aggressive behavior. Several months later, they were able to design a less stressful introduction to the regular class that was more successful.

Ritualistic habits, much like those associated with OCD, can consume the lives of autistic children. One family came to me for help with their seventeen-year-old because of the elaborate three-hour ritual necessary for him to eat a meal. Actual eating took only a few minutes, but the rest of his time was spent carefully lining up each item in rows from the upper left to the lower right in an order known only to him and changed with each meal. He would often demand an extra clean plate to move one piece of food so he could put another in its place, and then bring the first piece back onto the original plate. Any errors led to marked agitation and usually required him to start all over again. This routine had become so time-consuming that he could only eat one meal a day. In addition, this patient had elaborate touching rituals: Any time he went through a doorway, he had to touch different parts of the door in a specified order. Again, if he failed to do it just right, he would often have to start all over again. This sometimes meant his parents would drive him back to school, where he passed through his first door on the way home.

The day they came to see me, I witnessed a small portion of his parents' daily distress: It took him nearly half an hour to walk fifty feet from the waiting room to the examination room, because he had to go through three doorways. Either the anxiety of being in a new place or having new doorways to touch made the task especially difficult, because he had to start over many times. My one effort to persuade him to come through the doorways instantly changed him from a passive, self-preoccupied boy to a raging, aggressive, threatening young man large enough to give me pause. I immediately suggested, and the parents readily agreed to, a trial of the SSRI fluoxetine (Prozac). Irritability and tantrums are often responsive to SSRIs such as fluoxetine or sertraline (Zoloft). Within a month, his obsession had reduced by over 80 percent, with the only side effect being a slight interruption in his sleeping pattern that did not seem to interfere with his normal functioning. Although he remained autistic, his parents were thrilled not only with the reduced tension in the house but also with the many hours he now had free for other activities.

As you consider the possibility of medication, keep in mind that children can be particularly sensitive to both the benefits and the side effects of medications. I always counsel parents to "start low, go slow." Because medication use tends to increase over time, it is always best to start conservatively and use the lowest dose that proves effective. There are many possible types of medications to consider, with more coming on the market all the time, so it is possible that additional or alternative medications might be added later. The simpler the child's program is, the easier it is to guard against bad drug interactions.

Miracle Cures in the News

Autism is a debilitating disorder, so it is not surprising that parents are always searching for more effective treatments. They do not have to look far to find an abundance of stories of miraculous cures, either through diet-related regimens, behavioral-therapy techniques, or seemingly bizarre interventions like swimming with dolphins. These stories give some parents so much hope that they come into our autism clinic and are actually relieved when their child is diagnosed. Sadly, the number of autistic children who are actually "cured" of the core disorder remains distressingly low, and the waste of resources is enormous.

I fully support parents who come to me with a reasonable plan to try an alternative intervention. What works best, in my personal experience, is trying to achieve a diagnosis as early as possible and then address specific issues as they arise with established techniques. These popular alternative approaches persist, however, despite a dearth of research and often even in the face of substantive evidence against them.

One of these areas of attention has involved diet and intestinal dysfunction. Since autistic children tend to have a much higher incidence of gastrointestinal problems, proponents assert these children cannot tolerate certain types of food. These "allergies" are responsible for their autism, either directly or by letting in toxins that cause autism. It is interesting to note that these and similar claims over the years have initially asserted that the intervention "cures" autism, usually based on a single case. Over time, benefits will be reported, but typically the reports are far less dramatic than a cure. Later on, criticism that the treatment does not live up to its claims is dismissed, because autism is not so easily cured; yet the idea that "it must be doing something or so many people would not still be using it" still persists. Eventually, most of these treatments just fade away.

One of the more recent interventions involves secretin, a hormone produced by the pancreas. Based on the report of a dramatic recovery of one child who received a single injection of secretin as part of a work-up for chronic diarrhea, secretin rapidly became a must-have "cure," sometimes at well over a thousand dollars per injection. Despite having no idea how it could possibly have the reported effect, families and many experts in the field blazed ahead with enthusiasm. Gradually, controlled studies showed that a single secretin injection had none of the reported effects, yet advocates argued that was because it was the wrong kind of secretin and that it was foolish to expect a single injection to have a sustained effect. A drug company bought the rights for the gene for human secretin to make it available for study and began looking at administering multiple injections instead of just one. They also stopped focusing on a cure and began looking for improvement of any kind. Research ceased in 2004 due to a lack of evidence of substantial benefit. Even so, many are families still seeking secretin, just in case.

Parents have also begun seeking out chelation therapy, a treatment that strips the body of metals. Chelation therapy is used to detoxify people contaminated with metals through industrial accidents or environmental exposure. This approach, far from new but experiencing a recent resurgence, originates from the theory that autism is caused by the presence of heavy metals in the body, especially mercury-based preservatives found in childhood vaccines. Unfortunately, the drugs used in this treatment can have potentially serious side effects, including bone marrow and liver problems, because they also strip the body of necessary minerals, such as iron and zinc. Still, advocates say the treatment is worth the risk because it relieves some of autism's devastating symptoms, including lack of emotion and repetitive behaviors. This treatment got a boost when a toxicologist, treating his own son, testified before a congressional committee that nineteen of his thirty-one patients completely lost their autistic symptoms. This report was unpublished, and it is very possible this intervention will follow the same course as that of secretin treatments.

My advice to families is to use the same critical thinking with alternative interventions as with more conventional medications: Know your target symptoms, decide in advance how to best and most objectively mark changes in your child, and look out for side effects. Powerful interventions have the potential for powerful side effects. Remember, any time someone claims something is guaranteed to work and have no side effects, it is time to look elsewhere.

The Bottom Line

Children with developmental delays pose many challenges to their parents and to society. Most of the attention paid to these disorders relates to prevention, early detection, and interventions that maximize each child's ability to function. Medications have little to no role, especially in the early years.

However, children with these disorders are in no way protected from the other kinds of psychiatric disorders, and treatment of those conditions can be beneficial to their overall well-being. In addition, some children engage in such extreme behaviors that medication becomes essential for their own protection or for the protection of others. For those children, careful selection of an appropriate medication at the right dose can be enormously beneficial to them and to all around them.

PART THREE

Getting to Know Psychiatric Drugs

While professionals will evaluate a child and offer advice to the family about the appropriateness of medication, you, the parents, are ultimately the ones who will make the decision to medicate or not. As with many important decisions in life, we hope that the answer will be obvious and easy; unfortunately, it rarely is. I often tell parents that deciding to medicate a child is a bit like having sex: Whether it turns out to be a good or bad decision, you're never quite the same person afterward.

Jennifer was a sweet but incredibly disorganized seven-year-old whose parents were both pediatricians. She had a number of problems including a low but normal IQ, language difficulties, and some issues related to ADHD. After meeting with me several times to discuss whether medication might work for Jennifer, her parents decided to give medicine a try. We agreed to use methylphenidate (Ritalin) in the hope of a quick response, and because of our confidence in its safety. On the first day of the medication trial, Jennifer's parents called me in excitement and wanted to arrange a meeting as quickly as possible. When they came in, they said they were thrilled with the effect the medication had on Jennifer, and brought with them two samples of pictures she had colored. Off medication, Jennifer seemed to pick colors randomly; she scribbled hard, paying scant attention to staying in the lines, and stopped long before the picture was completed—what you might expect from a three- or four-year-old. On methylphenidate, her coloring was age-appropriate. The picture was no longer all purple, and she made reasonable color choices—trees now had green leaves and brown trunks, and she paid careful attention to staying within the lines and completing each picture.

Needless to say, coloring skills were not the barometer we had chosen for evidence of benefit, but we were all very pleased with Jennifer's new ability to stay on-task and to perform at an age-appropriate level. Over time, Jennifer continued to have problems with language as expected, but she had a far easier time working in school and at home than before.

Medicating a child doesn't always go as smoothly as it did with Jennifer. Beverly's parents brought their eight-year-old to see me because she had pervasive development disorder, a minor form of autism, and she also seemed unable to pay attention in class even when interested in the topic. After considerable debate, her parents and I decided on a trial of methylphenidate. Less than an hour after Beverly had taken the first dose, her parents urgently called me because her tongue was "twisted." When I saw her about a half hour later, I saw a reaction I had never seen before—or since. Beverly was in distress, but fortunately not in pain, and she was repeatedly sticking her corkscrew tongue in and out of her mouth. On a hunch, I gave her a small dose of a medication used to reverse a common reaction to some antipsychotic medications, and, within fifteen minutes, her twisted tongue returned to normal. Not surprisingly, we agreed to search again for ways to help Beverly without medication.

While drugs offer numerous benefits, they also all have the potential for side effects. **Ultimately, the decision to medicate is best made by answering the following questions:**

- Is the problem severe enough to warrant intervention?
- Have reasonable steps been taken to change the environment (i.e., a nightlight for a child who is afraid to use the bathroom, better supervision for the child with little impulse control, or a new classroom for a child who is not responding well to a teacher)?
- Have any appropriate nondrug therapies been explored?
- Has a meeting with school personnel been arranged to discuss programs for which the child may be eligible?
- What are the known advantages and disadvantages of the medication being recommended?
- How likely is it that the quality of life will improve as the result of medication?

- Are you sufficiently comfortable with the clinician recommending the medication? (You can always double-check a recommendation with your pediatrician.)

Ultimately, the decision you make must balance a number of factors. As you've read, many of the psychoactive medications being prescribed for children have not undergone long-term testing on children, which adds an unknown risk to your decision. For that reason, it's important for you and the medical professional involved to acknowledge when an intervention is not working. The child may be doing so poorly that you are ready to try anything for improvement, or perhaps the child's behavior is such that everyone is miserable. No matter the reason, something has happened that has made you ready for a new plan.

About Drug Testing

Most psychoactive drugs have not been studied for safety and effectiveness in children. With the exception of some older drugs "grandfathered" with research many years old, there are few drugs endorsed for children with psychiatric conditions. These are stimulants for ADHD, one antidepressant used to treat ADHD, and two drugs used to treat OCD.

No prescribed medication is marketed or sold in America without having undergone a rigorous approval process by the FDA. While requirements vary depending on the urgent need for a treatment, most medications must go through several years of trials before being approved. These trials generally involve what are called double-blind randomized-control studies. This means that neither the patients enrolled in the study nor the doctors conducting the research know which subjects are getting the medication being studied and which are getting a placebo (a look-alike capsule filled with an inactive ingredient). During the study, and for a period of time afterward, researchers monitor subjects for improvements and possible side effects. After a predetermined period, it is revealed who took the drug and who did not. Drug companies make major investments in these studies, so the FDA permits newly created drugs to be patented so generic copies can't be sold right away. This, in turn, affects the drug companies' ability to earn back their investments.

As discussed earlier, physicians often use medications off-label; that is, for reasons quite different from the purpose for which the FDA first endorsed their use. For example, nearly all the so-called "mood stabilizers" psychiatrists use to treat bipolar disorder and other problems with mood regulation first became available as anti-convulsants for seizure disorders. We use "antidepressants" to treat not only depression but also anxiety, OCD, bedwetting, and certain sleep disorders. This practice is especially common with children.

Drug testing is done on a condition-by-condition basis and for specific ages. For example, a new headache remedy might also ease joint pain, but if the study is focused on headaches in adults, then the FDA approval will only be for headache pain in that age range. As you read on, you will learn about medicines for other types of illnesses being used for mental disorders—the identification with the other illness simply explains what it received FDA approval for.

No matter how rigorous the testing, there are still flaws in the system. Because drug companies (understandably) want to get a medication to the marketplace if it has shown to be effective, approval is almost always given after a relatively short trial period of a limited number of subjects. However, it can take years to find out if there are benefits or drawbacks to long-term use of these medications, including serious side effects. The FDA has mechanisms for monitoring such post-marketing effects, but these results are not research-based, so sifting through and interpreting data can take time. One recent example is the newly revealed heart risks of Vioxx and similar pain medications. These medications had proven effective and were approved for pain management, but the long-term effects are only just becoming apparent. There are also new concerns about possible side effects of Adderall XR on the heart—concerns that so worried the Canadian government that they withdrew the drug from the market—yet the U.S. FDA considers the concern minor and not worthy of action.

Forty years ago, no one considered the possible downside of testing new drugs on children. The value of stimulants for ADHD first emerged from a study in which a pediatrician gave amphetamine to all of the boys in an orphanage and took note when the most hyper ones calmed down significantly. Attitudes toward medical testing on humans have changed since then, with children especially protected because they cannot properly assess the potential risk of participating. Understandably, many parents are reluctant to offer up their child as a guinea pig. Pharmaceutical companies also are reluctant to study children. The death of or serious injury to a child in a drug study would reflect very poorly on the drug company. This impasse leads to drugs being approved for those eighteen and older, which means they are then immediately used in children and adolescents, often in the hope that "newer is better."

This issue affects all types of medications for children, not just psychoactive drugs. It also clearly illustrates that children are not simply little adults. Their bodies metabolize medications differently, and because they are still growing, critical developmental processes are occurring. There is new concern that these developmental processes may be affected by medication. (My own brother was a child when tetracycline antibiotics first became available back in the late 1950s; he received tetracycline for an infection and still has stained teeth. The effect on tooth enamel wasn't apparent in clinical trials of adults or even in children until years later, when their permanent teeth began to come in severely discolored.)

Similarly, although stimulants have been used to treat children with ADHD since the early 1960s, we still are uncertain whether they have the long-term effect of reducing height. Their safety and efficacy for treating ADHD in adults is under investigation only now. Especially problematic are the rare, but serious, side effects that sometimes occur with any medication. These side effects may occur only once or twice out of hundreds of thousands or even millions of uses, like the little girl's curled tongue mentioned earlier. Identifying, let alone preventing, such effects is virtually impossible.

As a result, there is more information about the effects of older drugs on children simply because they've been in use longer. In sharp contrast, newer pharmaceuticals initially seem as good or better than older ones and less plagued with side effects, either because they really are safer or because of a lack of knowledge about them. This conundrum leaves physicians, patients, and parents with the troublesome choice of going with the known or the new.

How Physicians Learn About New Drugs

Physicians hear about new medications or new uses of old medications in a variety of ways. Pharmaceutical companies are eager to begin making profits as soon as the FDA endorses the use of a new drug, so they encourage rapid dissemination of information through presentations at professional meetings, company-sponsored education sessions by phone or on the Internet, and through "detailers" who meet with doctors to discuss the product. In addition, physicians often have local or even national networks of colleagues with whom they talk regularly and share their experiences with new medications.

Publications about the effects of medications appear in a range of professional journals. These reports can be as simple as a case history about an odd side effect or promising benefit in one or a small number of patients, or as complex as a full analysis of large-scale controlled trials with well-defined diagnoses and precise assessments of outcomes and side effects. Such studies can take decades to complete.

Sometimes doctors even hear about medications directly from their patients. Over the past few years, direct advertising from pharmaceutical companies to the general public through magazines, radio, TV, and the Internet has become a major information source for the public. Although I consider myself well-informed about psychoactive medications, parents have brought me new information about something they have found on the Internet, prompting me to consult more formal sources for additional information.

Getting Started

Here are some general rules about the use of medications:

- **Pick a time for your child to try a medication when nothing crucial is happening.** Don't start a new medicine during final exams or when the whole family is going on vacation. If the problems are occurring in school, don't try the medicine in the summer.

- **Make sure you have a good sense of the type and severity of symptoms you are targeting.** Consider making a chart to help you keep track.
- **Be aware that side effects often happen early, with benefits frequently kicking in later.** Be patient; if side effects continue to grow worse, speak up.
- **Give it time.** Make sure you have a sense how long it may take for a medication to take full effect. Some work in minutes; others can take weeks. Try one medication thoroughly before abandoning it and moving to another.
- **Don't hesitate to discuss concerns with your doctor.** If a behavioral change, good or bad, occurs, let the doctor know. If he or she understands what is bothering you, you can determine together if it might be medication-related.
- **Keep it simple.** Try medicines one at a time, and change dosage increases and decreases slowly.
- **Be prepared to experiment.** For most conditions, no one drug is guaranteed to work. Each patient must be evaluated individually, and his or her own age, medical issues, and personal circumstances must be taken into account. No matter how good or experienced the prescribing physician may be, there can still be reasons to make some changes.

Keeping Track

I strongly urge parents to keep records of their child's experiences with medications. This information may be relevant at some point in the treatment, so creating a paper trail, rather than relying on memory, is well worth the time.

Your record need not be elaborate—a simple notebook system is just fine. I ask parents to record when each new medication was started, the dose and times of administration, and apparent benefits and side effects. As memorable as a particular drug reaction may be, it can easily be forgotten in the months or years that follow, and at some point in the future this information may be quite significant. Your prescribing physician will be very appreciative of a first-hand report as well.

Timing

With disorders such as ADHD, you'll want to discuss with the doctor when your child should actually take the medication. Many parents only want to medicate for the span of the day when it's most important. Most families who turn to medication to treat ADHD have been urged to do so by schools, so achieving better focus during the day is usually the goal.

Getting out of the house in the morning is usually stressful for all households, but in

BRAND-NAME VS. GENERIC

If a generic drug exists for the medication being prescribed for your child, your insurance company will want you to purchase the generic form. In fact, many insurance companies won't pay for the brand-name drug if a generic one exists in the marketplace, or will insist you pay the difference in cost.

Will this be a problem for your child? The answer is almost universally no. Generic drugs must comply with rules set out the FDA, and these rules state that the active ingredient in the generic must be the bioequivalent to that of the brand-name drug. Therefore, if the medicine your child is taking has been made generically, he or she will be fine with the alternative drug. However, many parents find that generic alternatives don't work exactly like the brand-name one did. There may be differences in how quickly the drug begins to work or for how long. If you must make such a switch and believe your child is having a different reaction to the medication, notify your doctor to see if a change is needed.

families where ADHD is an issue, it can be all the more so. Parents may have to wake the child twenty to thirty minutes earlier than normal so the child can take the medication and function better in the morning. There is now a medication effective for ADHD called atomoxetine (Strattera) that has effects that carry over to the next day, potentially alleviating this problem.

For many disorders, the idea of using the medication only when it's most needed simply isn't feasible. For example, if a child has severe aggressive tantrums, the beginning of a tantrum is hardly a good time for your child to take a pill. Even if the child did agree, it would take up to thirty minutes for the pill to be absorbed, at which

point most tantrums are long over.

Most psychoactive drugs are best if taken at approximately the same time each day, so it's important to think about logical times for your child to take his or her medicine. Try to connect medication time with something that happens regularly in your day-to-day life. Sometimes it is best if the child is given medication upon waking. If a medication must be given twice daily, then you'll need to find two such times to connect with medicine-giving. Breakfast time at home is one such good opportunity, and a full stomach guards against nausea from any drugs for which that may be a possible side effect. Before bed is another good time, especially for medications that are sedating. Remember to also consider how you will administer medicine on the weekends.

These issues can be particularly difficult in divorced families where children may split their time between households. Even if both parents agree on their child taking medication, it can be a hassle to make sure that the pills and the child are in the same place. There is also the concern that one parent will recurrently "forget" or outright refuse to make sure the child takes the medicine. Certain kinds of medicines actually pose physical danger to the child if they are stopped and started abruptly, so such possible problems must be brought to the doctor's attention immediately.

Getting It Down

I have one absolute dictum: Pills never work if the child doesn't swallow them. Many children, and some adults, simply never learned to swallow pills. Make sure to discuss this issue with your doctor—an increasing number of medications are available in liquid form or in capsules that can be opened and sprinkled on food. Some pills, however, must be swallowed intact or are too bitter to swallow when crushed. Do not hesitate to make the doctor aware of such problems.

In Appendix A (page 256), I've listed some suggestions that parents have de-

vised to help their children get the medicine they need.

To Supervise or Not to Supervise?

So, if pills work only if the child takes them, how can you be sure a child is actually taking the medication prescribed?

I once had a family come to me for a consultation because the antidepressant their son had been taking for several years suddenly stopped working. The parents had him take his pills at breakfast and supper when they were sitting at the table together, so they were convinced he was getting the medicine. Fortunately, this medication can be measured in the blood, and a test showed no evidence of the medication in his system. I explained to the boy what the test showed and asked him directly how this could be. With chagrin, he admitted that several months earlier he had found a small hole in the central support of the family's old wooden table. The hole was just big enough for the pill to fit into, and he'd been depositing the pills in this crevice for some time. Sure enough, when the family removed the tabletop, they found about one hundred pills. I then spoke with the patient about why he decided to stop taking the medicine and found he was worried that he wouldn't be able to be sad because he was taking an antidepressant. Once I clarified that he was not taking medicine for that effect, he was willing to start it again and immediately regained its benefits.

Early in my career, I had another patient whose parents disagreed about pretty much everything, including whether their son needed to be on medication. About a month after beginning a medication trial, the father, who opposed his son being on medication but agreed to a trial, proudly proclaimed that it hadn't worked. I was curious about the fact that, even though the child was on a fairly high dose, he was experiencing no benefits but also no side effects. A blood test again revealed no trace of the medication. In discussing this, his parents explained that, to avoid embarrassing their son, they would hand him his pills each evening and let him go into the bathroom so he could take them in private. The mother casually mentioned that the toilet always flushed soon after he went in, but neither parent had thought anything about it. I then talked to the patient, who explained that he was sure the pills were poison. This led to a frank discussion with the patient and his parents about how the son was interpreting his parent's disagreements. Eventually, we conducted a trial and were able to get medication into him, with good results.

There is no easy answer as to whether to supervise a child while taking medications. In fact, there are several important aspects to the issue, including:

- **Safety.** These are powerful medications that should be taken as prescribed—no more or no less. If the child is too young or otherwise unable to understand that, then parents should retain control of administering medication. Similarly, a severely depressed or labile adolescent shouldn't be expected to resist the urge to overdose. If you are concerned about your child finding the medications unsupervised, be sure to store all medications in a locked cabinet or in an inaccessible spot.

- **Reliability.** A child with ADHD often has severe problems keeping track of routine tasks, and adding taking medication to those tasks may be asking too much. When stimulants only came in short-acting forms, schools would often blame the child for not remembering to stop playing during recess, go to the school nurse, and take the next dose. If the child could do that, he wouldn't need the medicine!

- **Motivation.** If a child is ambivalent about taking the medicine or might be tempted to do something else with it (i.e., trade it to a peer who promises to be his best friend for the day), then parents need to monitor the child.

- **Participation.** We want children and adolescents to have a sense of involvement in their treatment, and helping them feel at least partially responsible for taking their medication can help achieve that goal, as long as it actually leads to their getting the medication the way they should.

Teenagers are another story. We all know the temptations of adolescence, either from direct experience or from observing others. Many medications used for psychiatric disorders have little street value, but some do, especially stimulants. Furthermore, the actual "punch" of a medication, which may not be all that much, often has little to do with teen interest in trying it out. Both the physician and the parents need to be clear that prescribed medications should be used only for the person they are prescribed for, and that pills are for swallowing, not snorting or injecting.

I've had a number of patients who would never think of misusing their medications themselves but cannot resist the pressure from their peers. A lonely child with severe ADHD may find it tempting to trade his daily dose for the promise that someone will be his partner in gym class. The best parental defense against this possibility is awareness and a frank discussion of why not to share drugs with others, let along use drugs that someone else offers.

If you are worried your child might not be taking the medication, or if medication starts disappearing, talk to your doctor. Helping patients, especially adolescents, deal with their struggles to take medication is often the most important part of my work.

School attitudes toward medications are also important. The zero-tolerance policies that some schools have adopted can result in expulsion for carrying aspirin in your pocket, let alone a stimulant. If your child needs to take medication during the school day, make sure you know what the school policy is and follow its procedures.

Drug Interactions

Whenever possible, I try to keep the drug routine simple. Particularly with children, I prefer to find the proper medication rather than the proper mix of different drugs. Occasionally, it's necessary to add other drugs to a child's regimen, but with each additional drug comes the concern about complicating interactions. Most over-the-counter drugs are safe enough to give in combination with most psychoactive drugs. Cold and allergy medicines that contain antihistamines are exceptions, because they can intensify drowsiness in children who are taking sedating medications. Generally, there is no reason for concern, but it is always wise to check with your doctor.

Families confronting a mental disorder in a child sometimes feel desperate or helpless, and they may turn to herbal medicines or other types of nutritional supplements for help. Because the FDA does not monitor the safety and efficacy of these substances, manufacturers are not held to the same stringent standards for safety claims they may make in advertising. As a result, the bottles or the ads for the remedies make proclamations that have never been tested under the same types of clinical trials medications must undergo. A pervasive myth is that because these are natural substances, they must be safe. It is important to remember that arsenic and hemlock—both deadly poisons—also are natural.

Make sure to let the doctor know if you are giving any vitamins or herbal remedies to your child. They can have powerful interactions with prescribed medications.

Working with the School

Many parents are strongly ambivalent about involving their child's school in issues relating to medication, even when the problems are school-based. They fear that schools cannot maintain privacy, that teachers will treat their child differently because of the medication, and that information entered on the child's school record may have negative consequences later on. With rare exceptions, this has not been my experience, but I still try to work with parents to decide what is truly best for their child.

Sometimes teacher input is crucial. For instance, problems with inattention may manifest mostly in the classroom setting. Determining an optimal dose for a stimulant, then, becomes nearly impossible without teacher input. Still, teachers do not necessarily need to know all the details. I sometimes suggest that parents let a teacher know they are making some changes and ask her to provide feedback blindly, explaining that this is the best way to ensure that the changes they are making are really helping the child. As long as the information requested is not burdensome, most teachers are delighted to help.

As mentioned earlier, medications are seldom the only intervention needed for optimal treatment of most childhood mental disorders. Once you know how much benefit a child can receive from medications, it is time to begin thinking about how the school can provide additional assistance, if needed. This is also a good place to discuss what the school should know and how best to deal with the school officials.

Explaining Medication

Children have a right to know what is happening to them. Telling them that they are just taking a vitamin when in fact it's a

DEALING WITH YOUR OWN FEELINGS

Many parents have surprisingly intense feelings about giving a psychoactive medication to their child. Some years ago, a faculty member in my department asked me to see his college-age son, Jacob, for possible ADHD. Jacob had gotten above-average grades throughout high school but was about to fail his first year of college. Jacob had heard about ADHD in adults and told his father, a psychiatrist, he thought he might have it. It turned out that his grades in elementary and high school were primarily a reflection of the extraordinary time and structure his parents had given him. Even so, it was unclear how much his college grades reflected a lack of effort and self-motivation on his part as opposed to having ADHD. Frankly, the results of his trial of methylphenidate amazed me. Jacob still had poor study habits and hated to go to class, but his grades shot up to nearly all As and stayed there for the rest of his undergraduate education. More astonishing for me, however, was his parents' reactions. They felt intensely guilty for not having recognized and dealt with his ADHD years earlier, and their initial tendency to blame each other nearly broke up their twenty-three-year marriage. In the end, Jacob was fine, but I had to do a lot of work with his parents.

stimulant for their ADHD is apt to leave them confused and suspicious of adults. It can also lead to unfortunate occurrences such as the child taking "vitamins" to school to share with friends.

Like other topics parents must broach with their children, the level of detail varies with the child's age. A six-year-old may only need to know that he is taking medicine to help him focus better. Older children will probably have much more detailed questions such as why they have to take something that makes them feel "slowed down." The doctor should help explain the purpose of a medication to both the child and the parents. I often explain it

several times: to the child alone, to the parents alone, and then to all of them together. Since it can be tough to grasp sometimes, repetition can be a big plus.

Other parents worry that the medicine is for them and not their child, or they are so obsessed about possible side effects that they become nervous wrecks. Some feel so relieved about liking their child again that they feel guilty for their earlier feelings. Whatever feelings you may have, rest assured that you are not the first to have them. If they begin to interfere with your ability to provide the care your child needs or with your own mental health, talk to the doctor about how you are feeling.

Parent support groups also can be an excellent resource for helping acknowledge and cope with your reactions not just to medications but also to many other aspects of being the parent of a child with behavioral or mood issues.

Keeping Your Child in the Picture

Medication has the potentially powerful effect of changing how you see your child and interpret his behaviors. In an ADHD study I conducted, the relationship between parents and children who received methylphenidate actually worsened somewhat, even though the children improved in almost all other ways. I believe that adverse effect occurred because the medicine became the explanation for changes in behavior, either good or bad. If the child had a good day, it was because the medicine was working; a bad day meant the child forgot his pill or the dose needed to be increased. In short, the child has disappeared from the equation. Similar issues can arise for parents as their children go through puberty—is a particular behavior a normal part of adolescence, a result of the mental disorder, or a failure of medication?

All there is to do about this issue is simply warn parents about what can happen. Keep in mind that your child is far more than a test tube. She is going to have good days and bad ones, just like everyone.

Medication may change some behaviors, but antidepressants won't prevent normal feelings about a disappointing grade or the death of a pet, nor will stimulants keep a child from being bored with a dull teacher or sometimes hitting a sibling who is being a pest. Read books, talk to other parents, and meet with your child's doctor whenever you find yourself losing sight of the child who swallows the pills each day.

What to Tell Others

Several groups of people—siblings, other relatives, peers, teachers, day-care providers, and coaches, among others—may be directly affected by your child going on medication, so you'll need to give some thought as to what to say.

The first group of people you should speak to are those who most need the information. Grandparents or relatives who participate in a child's care will, of course, need to know about a new medication. They are less likely to be critical about this decision, perhaps because they are also very aware of the issues with which the family has been wrestling. It is possible, however, that some family members will insist the child just needs "more discipline" or is merely "being a kid."

Siblings are next. The last thing your child needs is to be taunted by brothers or sisters, so the more matter-of-fact you are, the better it will be for sibling relations. Trying to keep it a secret seldom works, so I usually recommend a straightforward explanation—the pills are important for their sibling's well-being. Any teasing that may arise should be dealt with the same way you deal with other sibling squabbles.

When it comes to sharing the information with in-laws, extended family members, and friends, parents usually start by telling a small circle of close relatives to test out what kinds of reactions they receive. One mother resisted putting her child on medication for months because of the reaction she was sure her sister would have. When she finally agreed to let her son start medication, he had a prompt positive response that led to general praise from family members regarding her improved parenting skills. Reluctantly, she admitted it was medication, not parenting, that had made the change. To her amazement, her sister then confided that her son had been on the same medication for several years.

One common question, especially with older children, is what they should tell their friends. There is no single right answer, but the issue is an important one that may require revisiting over time. A child with OCD may not want anyone to know about either the symptoms or the treatment; one with depression may be convinced that talking about needing

treatment will just drive everyone away. A child with ADHD may impulsively share, only to have it become yet another source of teasing. Children have a lot less privacy than we do; if a child has to take medication during a sleepover or during school, it will soon become common knowledge. You'll want to strategize with your child what he or she is comfortable saying.

Still, stigma about psychiatric disorders and medication treatment is all too real. In general, I encourage patients and their families to find a middle ground between lying and full disclosure. Parents can also monitor comments and reactions as they decide whom to inform. Perhaps even more important, I encourage parents to be open with their child and listen to how he or she prefers to handle the information.

Success—
More Than Medication

Medication alone is rarely the answer. If your child is going to start taking a medication, sit down with the prescribing physician, the therapist, or the school psychologist, and say, "What else should we be doing?" For example, the child on newly prescribed ADHD medication will still need help organizing schoolwork and can benefit from a structured method for doing homework. Children with Asperger's disorder will need parental guidance on developing proper social skills—they know they are awkward around other people, but they can't think of social remedies all by themselves. Evidence clearly shows that children with phobias typically do best with a combined approach, using medication to reduce anxiety and panic attacks and a behavioral approach that helps the child to face his fears so that they become less overwhelming. A child dealing with severe trauma may need medications to help with sleep and anxiety, but also needs therapy to help put past events into context.

Often, families who have been coping with a mental disorder can become somewhat dysfunctional—the demands of a child with additional physical or emotional needs take a toll on all family members. One goal of the physician will be to help the family right itself. Other siblings will benefit from some attention, and the child beginning treatment will actually do much better if tension in the household lessens. This additional "prescription" must be taken as seriously as the actual pills; medication alone is no substitute for the family and school working together to create a more comfortable environment for the child.

Just as the child needs to begin to experience small successes, so, too, does the family. Think of small steps to take toward accomplishing valuable lifestyle goals. While it may be a long time before all of you can meet Grandma for dinner at a fancy restaurant, you can focus on something easier to achieve: If a child can be good while you have lunch at a deli with outside tables, then you can eventually take on the challenge of a restaurant with table service. Many restaurants are family-friendly, but keep in mind that service can be slow—bring along something for the child to do, or plan to order and then let one adult take the child for a walk before the food arrives.

When Is a Drug No Longer Needed?

Essentially all of the medications currently available for psychiatric disorders are highly effective for reducing symptoms but do not affect the underlying problem. Thus, antidepressants can relieve depressive symptoms and even prevent the onset of a new episode of depression, but a single course of antidepressants does not permanently cure the disorder. On the other hand, development, an essential facet of childhood, sometimes can change a child's brain function or adaptive abilities so profoundly that earlier problems simply cease to be an issue. This has been best observed with ADHD: about one-third of children with severe ADHD at age eight will still have severe problems as an adult, while another third will be essentially symptom free.

How, then, do parents decide how long their child should stay on an effective medication? Sometimes medications need to be reevaluated because as the child grows older, the medication may cease to work or may begin to have unacceptable side effects. But suppose your child is doing wonderfully and has few or no side effects. What then?

My typical advice is to reassess the value of the medication periodically, especially after major transitions such as puberty or a move from one school setting to another. Several strategies can be appropriate, including taking a "summer holiday" from the medication or simply slowly lowering the dose for a period and monitoring for a return of symptoms. Even if medication needs to be continued, such professionally monitored experiments can help the child and parents be aware of what the medication is doing for them.

Going Off a Medication

Going off a medication can be as big a deal as starting it and must be treated with respect. Some medicines actually have withdrawal syndromes that can range from discomforting to physically dangerous. For example, abrupt discontinuation of mood stabilizers can result in seizures, or a child whose panic attacks have been well-controlled with an antidepressant may be devastated if the attacks return after abruptly stopping the medicine. The pace with which medicines can be stopped varies enormously, but it is important to schedule such a change with the child's doctor and to go over possible outcomes in advance.

The Bottom Line

Sometimes generic information like the information provided in this chapter fails to stick in your memory, because it is not something that you can immediately apply to your life. So don't worry about all the details here, because the following chapters are what you have been waiting for. You might read all of them, or only the ones that pertain to your child. After you read these medication-specific chapters, consider skimming this chapter again. You will probably find that some points make more sense once you have a specific disorder and medication in mind.

Chapter 8

Antidepressants

· ·

When I entered the field of child psychiatry in the mid-1980s, antidepressants seemed to be the answer to almost any problem that plagued mentally ill children. Imipramine (Tofranil), a tricyclic antidepressant, was reportedly useful for depression, anxiety, ADHD, school phobia, OCD, bulimia, conduct problems, and even bedwetting! Accumulating evidence seemed to attest to the relative safety of this class of medications, and researchers and clinicians alike kept looking for new uses. While some were troubled by the fact that there was no conclusive evidence of efficacy, particularly in treating depression, most felt that this pointed to the difficulty in research design and not a problem with the medications themselves.

During the following years, acceptance of antidepressant use continued to grow, especially as new generations of less-toxic antidepressants became available. Finally, in the late 1990s, more than one well-performed study demonstrated that one antidepressant, fluoxetine (Prozac), was safe and effective for treating depression in children and adolescents, apparently affirming what many clinicians had long believed. Prescription rates of antidepressants for all ages ballooned. In mid-2004, a congressional hearing on prescription drugs noted that one in every six children in the U.S. was being prescribed an antidepressant.

I have been in the uncomfortable position of both encouraging the use of antidepressants for serious childhood illnesses and cautioning against blind optimism about their safety. The latter was not a matter of extraordinary prescience on my part—public confidence in these medications was known to be thin. In the late 1980s, clinicians reported the sudden deaths of five children over a span of several years that may have resulted from use of an antidepressant called desipramine (Norpramin). Uncertainty about the causes of those deaths plus the introduction of new, seemingly safer classes of antidepressants rapidly led to abandonment of the older medications even before any real information about how well these newer medications worked in young patients became available.

Events of the past few years, often chronicled in newspapers and news magazines, suggest that we are in the midst of another major change. In 1999, after the Columbine massacre, reporters learned that at least one of the perpetrators had been taking an SSRI, which is a fluoxetine-like antidepressant. Along with many of my colleagues, I was called upon by the media to provide a quote suggesting that the drug "made him do it."

In 2004, the defense for a South Carolina boy who killed his grandparents when he was twelve was based on the proposition that he was "involuntarily intoxicated" by sertraline (Zoloft) and therefore not responsible for his actions. Although the jurors did not find this a credible explanation and convicted the boy of murder, this illustrates how these medications are being portrayed in the media.

That same year, the British FDA grew alarmed at preliminary results of a study of paroxetine (Paxil) for treating anxiety in adolescents. They noted that some of the subjects taking the drug reported having thoughts of hurting themselves, and a few even made one or more suicide attempts, although none succeeded. The British government halted the study and banned the use of paroxetine in young patients with anxiety. The U.S. FDA reacted by sending a letter to all U.S. physicians strongly discouraging the use of paroxe-

tine for any purpose in younger patients. It then convened a group of experts to review the safety of all antidepressants in children and adolescents, followed by a reassessment of all available data from clinical trials with young subjects. The report concluded that, on average, about 1.5 to 2 percent of patients taking a placebo reported having suicidal thoughts or making suicide attempts, compared to 3.5 to 4 percent of patients taking one of the antidepressants under study. There were no completed suicides in any of the studies. Although the difference was not statistically significant—that is, the difference is quite possibly a result of chance—the FDA decided that all antidepressants should carry what is called a "black box" warning about the possible danger of increased suicidal tendencies.

These findings certainly are worrisome—a 100 percent increase in risk is nothing to dismiss lightly. On the other hand, perhaps the degree of concern need not be all that great. Suicidal thoughts are actually quite common, even among normal adolescents. Some studies have reported that 25 percent or more of teenagers have thoughts of self-harm sometime during adolescence; fortunately, the vast majority take it no further. Also, many of the subjects in these studies were depressed, and clinicians have long known that depressed patients who are beginning

ANTIDEPRESSANTS USED IN CHILDREN AND ADOLESCENTS

Drug	Typical Dose (mg/day)	Doses (per day)
TRICYCLIC ANTIDEPRESSANTS (TCAs)		
clomipramine (Anafranil)	25–150	2
desipramine (Norpramin)	25–250	2
imipramine (Tofranil)	25–250	2
notriptyline (Pamelor)	10–150	2
SELECTIVE SEROTONIN REUPTAKE INHIBITORS (SSRIs)		
citalopram (Celexa)	10–40	1
escitalopram (Lexapro)	5–20	1
fluoxetine (Prozac)*	10–100	1
fluvoxamine (Luvox)	25–200	1–2
paroxetine (Paxil)	5–40	1
sertraline (Zoloft)	25–150	1
OTHER ANTIDEPRESSANTS		
bupropion (Wellbutrin)	75–450	1–2
duloxetine (Cymbalta)**	20–60	2
mirtazapine (Remeron)**	15–60	1
trazodone (Desyrel)	25–600	1
venlafaxine (Effexor)	25–150	1–2

*FDA-endorsed for use in children and adolescents

**few to no studies of safety and efficacy in children

to respond to treatment sometimes go through a period of increased suicidal risk before they have fully recovered. Even if the risk is accurate, depression is not a trivial condition. It is clearly related to marked increases in suicidal risk, so failure to treat the disorder may pose even greater risks for the patient.

What does this mean for you as a parent considering using an antidepressant for your child? You've already read that no medicines are completely safe, and there is much left that is still unknown. Weigh the problems your child is experiencing, to the extent they are known, against the risks of medications and make the best judgment you can. Even more importantly, if you decide to try a medication, watch for adverse effects of any kind, and don't hesitate to speak up about any concerns you have.

In general, despite shifting public attitudes about antidepressants, you'll find that professionals still are using antidepressants for a wide range of disorders and behaviors (see table on reasons for using antidepressants in children) with considerable confidence. Especially the newer antidepressants are remarkably well tolerated, and have a low risk of serious toxicity even with deliberate overdoses. At present, however, many pediatricians are reluctant to prescribe them because the required monitoring is more intense than

they usually prefer. Do not be surprised if you need to find another child and adolescent psychiatrist to work with you if this is the class of medications your child needs.

How They Work

All antidepressants are thought to work the part of the brain called the hypothalamus. Nearly all of the effective antidepressants work to increase the activity of two neurotransmitters, serotonin or norepinephrine, and many affect both. The most common mechanism that antidepressants affect is called neuronal reuptake. Neurotransmitters work at synapses, the points in the brain where nervous impulses travel from one neuron to another. These synapses have "transporters" that collect neurotransmitters after they have carried their information and return them to storage vesicles, where they wait to be released again. Blocking those reuptake mechanisms causes the neurotransmitters to remain in the synapse longer, increasing the intensity and duration of their action.

Despite this knowledge, one of the great mysteries of psychiatry is how antidepressants work. They do increase neurotransmitter activity, but that is an immediate effect. Why, then, do antidepressants take two to four weeks, if not longer, to work? It it thought that there is a cascade effect of some kind, with the chronic elevation of neurotransmitter leading to unknown changes in the neuron that results in the antidepressant effect. Decades of studies in depressed individuals of all ages, as well as a wide range of animal models, have yet to yield a convincing answer. When it is found, there may be a whole new array of possibilities for different types of antidepressants.

It is also unclear why antidepressants work for such a wide range of seemingly disparate disorders. Occasionally an argument arises that all these disorders are linked somehow. It is equally possible, and in my opinion more likely, that it reflects our limited understanding of the many ways in which these complex compounds affect brain activity.

Tricyclic Antidepressants

One of the oldest groups of antidepressants, tricyclic antidepressants (TCAs) are closely related chemically and have a core structure of three rings, hence the name. All inhibit both norepinephrine and serotonin reuptake, although to differing degrees. As mentioned earlier, imipramine was the first antidepressant studied in children, beginning in the 1970s and 1980s. It was initially used for depression and rapidly thereafter for ADHD, anxiety, and many other conditions. Researchers chose to study it because it was already being used in children as a treatment for enuresis (bedwetting), so clinicians had some experience with dosage and safety issues. These drugs were widely prescribed but are scarcely used now for several reasons, including concerns about safety that arose in the late 1980s as well as the introduction of newer, safer antidepressants. They are still used intermittently for bedwetting and for certain chronic pain syndromes.

Although many children and adolescents tolerated TCAs remarkably well, they have drawbacks. As little as a week's supply of the medication, taken in deliberate or accidental overdose, can be lethal, causing the heart to stop beating properly. Even regular doses can affect the electrical conduction system of the heart and also produce unpleasant side effects such as severe dry mouth, constipation, blurry vision, and dizziness from lowered blood pressure with sudden changes of position. They can also increase the risk of seizures in vulnerable patients. They require the monitoring of blood concentrations to ensure the correct dosage, because individual dosages vary widely and change, even for the same individual, on the basis of pubertal status. Regular EKG monitoring is also recommended, because of concerns about the heart.

Research has failed to show that TCAs are effective for depression, but, ironically enough, it did compile fairly convincing evidence of benefits for a variety of other disorders.

Selective Serotonin Reuptake Inhibitors

The release in the U.S. of fluoxetine (Prozac) in 1986 produced wide ripples throughout all of psychiatry and medicine. Here, at last, was an antidepressant that was safe and effective at a wide range of possible doses and was unlikely to cause death even with massive overdoses. It required no monitoring, seemed generally well-tolerated with far fewer side effects than TCAs, and clearly worked for depression, OCD, and probably many other disorders. It became a best-selling medication worldwide, and outsold all other medications of any type for a number of years.

Not surprisingly, the success of a medication that worked specifically on serotonin reuptake led pharmaceutical companies to seek and eventually market other drugs that worked similarly (see table on antidepressants used in children and adolescents). Each found an eager market, and the reasons for prolonged use of this class of medications continued to grow at an amazing pace. A few years ago, the top five most-prescribed medications in the pharmacy of the general medical hospital at the University of California, San Francisco, where I work, were all SSRIs. In like fashion,

child and adolescent psychiatrists and other physicians who treat children and adolescents for mental disorders also came to rely on these medications, with mixed results. For example, ADHD is not very responsive to SSRIs, even though many other disorders and conditions are (see table on reasons for using antidepressants).

Side Effects

SSRIs differ somewhat among themselves with regard to possible side effects. For example, fluoxetine and sertraline (Zoloft) are both energizing and often cause insomnia, while paroxetine (Paxil) and fluvoxamine (Luvox) are more likely to be calming and even sedating. Clinicians have learned to prescribe an SSRI on the basis of such likely side effects.

Other common side effects of the SSRIs include agitation, oversedation, and rashes, especially for fluoxetine. One condition, called akithesia, has been of considerable interest. Some patients, especially when starting an SSRI or after a dose increase, begin to experience a sense of unease and physical restlessness. Some have speculated that these feelings, especially when not recognized as a side effect of the medication, may be one of the reasons patients have suicidal thoughts early in treatment. A more chronic problem for both men and women can be reduced sexual drive and problems reaching orgasm.

Perhaps not surprisingly, clinicians were slow to discover this side effect in teenagers both because adolescents are unlikely to volunteer this information and neither parents nor physicians thought to ask.

Efforts to establish safety and efficacy of SSRIs for disorders such as depression and anxiety has led to results that prompted the FDA to issue warnings about suicide for all antidepressants. Although this has produced some dampening in enthusiasm, this class of medications continues to have widespread use.

Other Antidepressants

A number of antidepressants do not fit well into either of the above categories. Several are non-TCAs that inhibit both norepinephrine and serotonin reuptake: mirtazapine (Remeron), venlafaxine (Effexor), and the newer duloxetine (Cymbalta). None of these medications have been extensively studied in young patients. Like the SSRIs, they seem largely well-tolerated, with few major safety concerns in terms of physical effects.

Another drug, trazodone (Desyrel), is intriguing because it does not directly affect norepinephrine or serotonin reuptake, and the manner in which it works remains unclear. It became available in the early 1980s, but never gained popularity as an antidepressant because it is highly sedating and may be less effective than many others drugs. I prescribe it primarily—and almost exclusively—for children with developmental disorders who have trouble sleeping. It is also unusual in that it can cause priapism (a sustained erection), a rare side effect that is a medical emergency.

Bupropion (Wellbutrin) was released a few years after fluoxetine, and it too has a novel mode of action thought to relate to increased dopamine activity. It appears to have benefits for ADHD as well as for depression, but studies in children and adolescents are quite limited. Part of the obstacle lies in the history of the drug. In the early 1980s, the pharmaceutical company presenting research to the FDA for bupropion's release in the U.S. was eager to study its possible uses in younger patients. It sponsored trials for both ADHD and bulimia, but they ran into problems with the trials for bulimic patients because a proportion suffered seizures. This delayed the introduction of bupropion until several years after fluoxetine flooded the market. That experience may well have discouraged other companies from vigorously pursuing medications for use in children and adolescents.

A last broad category of antidepressants are called monoamine oxidase inhibitors (MAOIs). These drugs are about as old as the TCAs, and work through a different mechanism, blocking a metabolic enzyme that inactivates both norepinephrine and serotonin reuptake. These medications never had widespread use, even in adolescents and far less so for children, because they can interact with a variety of common foods, producing a dangerous and potentially fatal elevation in blood pressure.

Dosage

Most antidepressants have similar levels of response, with some exceptions. Thus, if the target disorder is ADHD, an SSRI is unlikely to work but several other antidepressants might. For many disorders or behaviors, the family and physician can choose a medication based on which are least frightening to the family, which medications the doctor has used the most, or what has worked (or not worked) for other family members. I also want to consider how best my patient will respond to some of the known side effects. For example, I may suggest fluoxetine or sertraline for a lethargic, depressed adolescent who sleeps

---

REASONS FOR USING ANTIDEPRESSANTS
IN CHILDREN AND ADOLESCENTS

DISORDERS

> Anxiety disorders
> Attention-deficit/hyperactivity disorder (ADHD)*
> Bulimia
> Enuresis (bedwetting)**
> Major depression
> Obsessive-compulsive disorder (OCD)***
> Post-traumatic stress disorder (PTSD)

SEVERE BEHAVIORS

> Uncontrollable agitation, aggression, or rage
> Labile mood with temper outbursts
> Obsessive behaviors
> Self-injurious or mutilating behaviors, such as cutting

*only some antidepressants, including TCAs and bupropion
**only TCAs
***only SSRIs

NOT JUST FOR DEPRESSION

At age nine, Henrietta's life was falling apart. Despite having an IQ of 135, she was convinced she was stupid and was doing her best to get kicked out of school, which she hated. Testing showed that she had a nonverbal learning disability (NVLD). Her verbal IQ was about 150, but her nonverbal or performance IQ was closer to 110. As is true for many children with NVLD, Henrietta hated surprises or transitions; unless parents and teachers were extremely careful in preparing her for a change, she would often completely fall apart, starting what could be a prolonged meltdown with kicking, screaming, even head banging. She had enormous problems with peers because she simply couldn't understand nonverbal cues, such as gestures and body positioning, from them. She also had trouble settling down at night, often demanding that her parents come in several times over the course of an hour to reassure her that no one was in her room or trying to break into the house.

We started Henrietta on 5 mg of paroxetine at bedtime, which had no effect at all. Increasing the dose to 10 mg four days later promptly improved her ability to fall asleep. Over the course of the next several weeks, she, her parents, and her teachers all noticed that Henrietta was mellower, better able to transition from one task to another, and far less likely to fly into a rage. She began to work with a counselor to help her deal with her self-esteem issues and to plan other ways of coping with change. A social skills group helped with her peer problems, but she still tended to do better with adults than with children her own age. Two years after starting the medication, Henrietta began to enter puberty. Because she was growing rapidly, we increased her dose to 20 mg each evening, but she began to complain of daytime sedation, so we dropped the dose back to 10 mg, which worked fine.

too much, since these drugs tend to decrease sleep and enhance energy. For someone who has trouble getting to sleep and is already agitated, I am more likely to chose mirtazapine (Remeron) or paroxetine, which are more calming and sedating.

It is generally better to start with a low dose and build up slowly over several weeks as the patient becomes accustomed to the medication. However, because these medications all take several weeks to begin working, especially for depression, families often ask to get the child up to a "therapeutic dose" as quickly as possible. With many patients, a reasonable compromise is to start at about half a usual dose and double it four to seven days later.

Actual dosage requirements differ for different drugs, individuals, and conditions. Typically, anxiety responds better to relatively lower doses; depression, bulimia, and probably ADHD to somewhat higher doses; and OCD to relatively high doses. In my experience, patients with developmental delays tend toward the extremes: Some respond well to and only tolerate low doses, while others require doses in the top range. Frequently, medication response is similar across different medications, so a sensitive child will probably do best on low doses of most medications. For some antidepressants, especially the TCAs, children generally require dosages based on their weight and are far higher than adults need or can even tolerate. This is because children metabolize medications more rapidly than adults do. These types of differences underscore the importance of working with a doctor who knows how to use psychoactive medications in children.

Most antidepressants are relatively long-acting, so taking the medication once or twice a day produces a steady effect. When twice-daily dosing is recommended, it is almost always to minimize side effects, not to improve benefits. In general, side effects worsen as levels of the medication in the blood increase, so spreading out the dose can reduce side effects. An increasing number of antidepressants now come in sustained-release preparations that produce that same result with only one daily dose.

Frequency

Unlike stimulants, antidepressants must be taken every day. It's okay to miss an occasional dose (although I have seen children's symptoms quickly return even when they miss just one day) but effective use of these medications requires consistent administration. For similar reasons, it makes no sense to use an extra pill to help your child through an especially hard day—antidepressants simply don't work that way.

When to take the medication depends largely on the side effects one wants to use or avoid. A medication that may cause insomnia is usually given as early in the morning as possible, while a sedating antidepressant is best taken just before bedtime. Some medications cause stomach upset that may be eased if taken with meals. I encourage doctors, patients, and families to experiment and find a time that works for them and produces the fewest problems.

As a rule, the side effects of antidepressants occur early and benefits late. Patients may need encouragement to continue taking the medication during those days or weeks, but patients and families also need to feel free to express any concerns. Those at risk for developing a manic response to an antidepressant tend to do so in the second or third week after getting to a therapeutic dose. Possible increased suicidal thoughts also occur early, usually in the first ten to fourteen days. I will typically have contact with a patient at least weekly during the first few weeks, preferably in person but certainly by phone. I will want to see them as soon as possible if side effects emerge or other unexpected changes occur.

Going Off an Antidepressant

Assuming the antidepressant works for the target disorder or behavior, the next hard decision is how long to keep using it. For depression, anxiety, bulimia, and other disorders that have a waxing and waning course, at least nine to twelve months of good functioning is usually recommended before trying to taper off the medication. I typically suggest a slow decrease over several months in hope that, even if we still need to continue the medication, a lower dose may work just as well. With ADHD, OCD, and severe recurrent anxiety or depression, ongoing antidepressant use may be the best course, checking in at critical developmental periods such as postpuberty and post-high school or college to determine continued need.

The Bottom Line

Antidepressants have become the main-stay of child psychopharmacology. They work for a variety of conditions, seem relatively safe with no known long-term adverse consequences, have little to no abuse potential, and require minimal medical monitoring. It is hardly surprising, then, that their use has skyrocketed over the past two decades. Unfortunately, it is also not surprising that at least some of that increase has been poorly considered and maybe even ill-advised.

Broadly speaking, antidepressants cure nothing but can make life markedly better when used appropriately. When I was a child—and the practice continues today—physicians used antibiotics with similar abandon. My pediatrician gave me a penicillin shot at least once each year when I had a high fever and cough. These symptoms were almost certainly signs of a cold or flu, for which antibiotics are useless. Eventually, I developed a fierce rash after one such shot, eliminating the option of using penicillin for the rest of my life.

One argument is that if a medication is safe and there is no concrete way of knowing on whom and for what disorder it will work, then why not try it empirically to see who benefits? The counterargument is that assuming every problem can be solved with a medicine and that even safe medications, when used widely enough, will begin to reveal their dark sides. Again, my position is somewhere in the middle. I find it hard to countenance rigidly withholding a trial of medication because something bad might happen, but I also shy away from the more cavalier approach of, "Just take these pills for a few weeks and let me know if you like them."

Deciding to take a medication—any medication—should start with having an identifiable problem that seems more than transient and is interfering with normal functions. This medication should alleviate the problem with known side effects sufficiently mild or infrequent enough to be less worrisome than the problem it is treating. Finally, you need a system for monitoring both benefits and side effects so that, good or bad, you can decide at the end of the trial what the medication has accomplished and whether you should continue it.

Chapter 9

Antipsychotic Drugs

Antipsychotics are among the most versatile and poorly understood class of medications that child and adolescent psychiatrists have in their therapeutic arsenal. Also called "neuroleptics" or "major tranquilizers," all of the members of this family of medications produce profound changes not only in thinking processes but also in the general level of physical and emotional arousal. Their primary use is for those with psychotic thinking; that is, for those who have begun hearing voices, seeing things that aren't there, or experiencing other impairments in their ability to process information. Beyond that, however, these medicines are used as last resorts for severe ADHD, OCD, and overwhelming anxiety, as well as for behavioral problems such as self-injurious behaviors or recurrent aggression toward others.

Psychosis is a condition caused by any number of illnesses (e.g., schizophrenia, bipolar disorder, or severe depression), and it results in the person losing contact with reality. During a psychotic episode, people may experience delusions (thinking that they are stronger than a superhero or that they can fly), hallucinations (hearing voices or seeing or feeling things that are not there), and thought disturbances (impaired logic or inability to stay on topic). In addition, they may become angry for no apparent reason, spend a lot of time by themselves or in bed, or sleep during the day and stay awake at night; many experience a decreased interest in daily activities and a blunting of their emotions.

Antipsychotic medications work to minimize symptoms of delusions and hallucinations or disorganized thinking. The first antipsychotic medications were introduced in the 1950s and were initially created to relieve symptoms of schizophrenia; though they are successful at this, there are very definite side effects.

William, the thirteen-year-old son of a psychiatrist in our community, had been doing extremely well in all aspects of his life until about a month before he came to see me. He had entered puberty about six months earlier and, after a growth spurt, had become interested in participating in basketball at his school. Then, quite abruptly and without any clear external causes, William began to grow fearful about going to basketball practice. At first he refused to say why, but his parents noticed that he was sleeping less, was having considerable difficulty getting his homework done, and seemed withdrawn at home. They also observed that he'd begun

---

USING ANTIPSYCHOTICS

Tony was a seven-year-old with autism and moderate mental retardation. He was in a loving home and a good school, but Tony could not handle even the smallest of surprises. A rapid transition from one task to another or a sudden noise, such as the siren of a passing ambulance, could set him off. Between three and ten times a week, such a disturbance would provoke a tantrum that involved severe aggression, usually against whoever happened to be closest to him at the time. Some of his outbursts included biting hard enough to break the skin; another violent incident sent one teacher to the emergency room because of a blow to her eye. Alternatively, he might attack himself, repeatedly slamming his closed fist against the side of his head as hard as he could or throwing himself against the wall or onto the floor until someone successfully stopped him.

Behavioral interventions were completely unsuccessful in preventing these tantrums. After talking with Tony's parents about the relative risks and benefits of the new antipsychotics over the older ones, they elected to use an older one, haloperidol (Haldol). An initial dose of 0.25 mg a day had no discernable side effects. Slow increases over several weeks eventually led to a dose of 0.25 mg each morning, 0.25 mg at noon, and 0.5 mg at night. At that level, Tony remained alert and aware of activities around him but became far more flexible, able to ignore outside disruptions to a degree never before possible. His parents and teachers were delighted. About two weeks into treatment, he had some muscle stiffness because of the medication, so a small dose of a second medicine, benztropine (Cogentin), was added to treat that. Several months later, the benztropine was stopped. However, even a small decrease in haloperidol led to renewed agitation, so dosage was maintained.

Over the next twelve years, Tony stayed on haloperidol without other problems, needing occasional increases to compensate for his increasing size. Efforts to reduce the dose every few years were all met with worsening behavior, until his late teens. At that point, Tony was working in a sheltered workshop (a workplace designed for adults with developmental disorders) in a group home. Gradual decrease of the haloperidol over two months led to no notable change, so he stopped medication altogether and has not required medication for the past several years.

---

to close his curtains and lock his door as soon as he came home, something he'd not done before. Eventually, William confided to his parents that he had been hearing people jeering at him while he was at basketball practice. At first he thought it was someone else on the team, but he could never catch the person doing it. Then, the same thing began happening at home, even when no one was around. He asked his parents to help him search for the speakers. They did, but their failure to find any just confirmed, from William's point of view, how clever the person harassing him was.

When I first met with William, he was confused and fearful. He agreed to speak with me only because I was a friend of his mother's, but he gradually grew comfortable enough to tell me about the voices and his fears. By that time, he'd begun to explain what was happening to him as the result of having special skills as a basketball player that made everyone else on the team envious. He also found that he needed only a few hours of sleep each night and had begun a number of ambitious projects, each dropped in favor of the next.

Because William was so disturbed and agitated, we started him on a low dose of an antipsychotic, in his case risperidone (Risperdal). He slept through the night for the first time in over a week; over the next few days, his thoughts began to clear and the voices went away. Still confused, he became incredulous about what had been happening to him, soon "forgetting" many of the details. Once his worst symptoms dissipated, he and his family agreed that he had a manic episode that was caught fairly early. He stayed on risperidone while starting on lithium, because he did not want to take any chance of having his symptoms return. Once he was on a therapeutic dose of lithium, we tapered the risperidone, and he has continued to do fine.

How They Work

Antipsychotics are prescribed to children and adolescents for two broad reasons: to treat a specific disorder or to control behaviors that are otherwise unacceptable (see table on reasons to use antipsychotics). In my experience, as much as we might wish it otherwise, the latter is a far more common reason than the former.

As implied by the name, antipsychotics reverse or at least reduce the major signs and symptoms we associate with psychosis, regardless of the underlying cause. This ability, first noted in the early 1950s in adults with schizophrenia, is one of the cornerstones of modern-day psychopharmacology. The precise mechanism by which they accomplish this effect remains a mystery, although all effective

ANTIPSYCHOTICS USED IN CHILDREN AND ADOLESCENTS

Drug	Typical Dose (mg/day)	Doses (per day)
TYPICAL (first generation)		
chlorpromazine (Thorazine)	25–400	1–4
fluphenazine (Prolixin)	0.25–5	1–4
haloperidol (Haldol)*	0.25–10	1–4
perphenazine (Trilafon)	2.5–24	1–4
pimozide (Orap)*	0.25–10	1–4
thiothixene (Navane)	0.5–30	1–4
thioridazine (Mellaril)	25–400	1–4
trifluoperazine (Stelazine)	1–10	1–4
ATYPICAL (second generation)		
aripiprazole (Abilify)	2.5–20	1–2
olanzapine (Zyprexa)	2.5–20	1–4
quetiapine (Seroquel)	25–800	1–4
risperidone (Risperdal)*	0.25–8	1–4
ziprasidone (Geodon)*	20–160	1–2

*demonstrated benefit for motor tic disorders such as Tourette's disorder

antipsychotics block the receptor for dopamine in the brain, and the relative potency (the doses of each drug needed to obtain a comparable benefit) of the antipsychotics correlates remarkably well with their potency as receptor antagonists, or blockers. How altering dopamine activity in the brain can exert this profound effect on brain function remains an active area of research.

The effect of antipsychotics on tic disorders such as Tourette's disorder has also been known for many years. Again, the blocking of a dopamine receptor seems to be the underlying mechanism that makes the drug effective. Different parts of the brain have different kinds of dopamine receptors, and tic disorders respond to antipsychotics that strongly affect one particular type of dopamine receptor. As a result, some drugs work quite well for this disorder, while others have little to no benefit.

Of recent interest has been the use of the atypical antipsychotics as the primary treatment for bipolar disorder. Researchers now have established their benefits in adults to the satisfaction of the FDA, and studies in adolescents with bipolar disorder are underway. The initial impetus for such studies was the belief that antipsychotics would be easier to use and potentially safer than more classic mood stabilizers, most of which are anticonvulsants. Emerging concerns about the side effects of atypical antipsychotics require a reassessment of relative risks.

The mechanisms through which antipsychotics improve other behaviors are not well understood but almost certainly involve a number of different effects on the brain. Both animal and human studies have repeatedly shown that antipsychotics markedly alter perception of and response to anxiety-inducing situations, leading to the concept of major tranquilizers. Although sedation may play a role in this effect, the change is much more than a matter of drowsiness. The impact seems to relate to both the assessment of the threat and the need to respond to that threat. Similarly, antipsychotics reduce repetitive behaviors, overall physical activity, and impulsive behaviors. Again, underlying mechanisms for these effects are poorly understood.

The goal, with antipsychotics in particular, is to use the least amount of medication possible to manage symptoms effectively, because most of the side effects that patients and parents find hard to tolerate are dose-dependent. For control of nonspecific symptoms, finding a medication the child can tolerate and then identifying the right daily dose and the time of distribution of doses over the day is the main focus. As with drug treatments for other physical illnesses, many patients with severe mental illnesses may need to try several different antipsychotic medications before they find the one or the combination that works for them.

Choosing an Antipsychotic

Typical (First-Generation) Antipsychotics

The success of the first antipsychotic medication, chlorpromazine (Thorazine), for treating schizophrenia in the early 1950s led to an intense and successful search for other chemicals with similar properties. By the late 1970s, physicians had their choice of over fifteen antipsychotics with different chemical structures and a fairly wide range of potencies and side effects (see table on antipsychotics used in children and adolescents). Since research showed that equivalent doses of all the antipsychotics had similar benefits (especially for psychosis) and had similar or identical short- and long-term side effects, the art of using antipsychotics lay mainly in choosing one on the basis of side effects, such as sedation, and how activated or slowed patients were on them.

With children and adolescents, research on the use of typical antipsychotics was sparse, at best. The most child-specific research involved using antipsychotics to treat behavioral disturbances in autistic children, and that research focused largely on the drug haloperidol. Most clinicians ended up using either haloperidol, which is fairly potent and nonsedating but produces other acute side effects or thioridazine or chlorpromazine, both of which are of lower potency and more sedating.

One of the biggest concerns about these first-generation antipsychotics was a potential long-term side effect called tardive dyskinesia (TD), a largely involuntary rhythmic movement of parts of the body. TD appears in about 15 to 20 percent of individuals taking atypical antipsychotics, usually over several years, and any of the atypical antipsychotics are equally as likely to cause it. TD can occur in anyone and is not clearly related medication dosage or length of treatment. Worst of all, it was untreatable until quite recently.

The risk of an effect like TD was difficult to deal with when one was treating adults with severe psychoses. It was even more worrisome when treating children for less clear diagnoses. It caused most physicians and parents to view antipsychotics as drugs to be used only as a last resort and maybe not even then.

Atypical (Second-Generation) Antipsychotics

The use of antipsychotics changed markedly in the late 1980s, when researchers discovered a new compound, clozapine (Clozaril). Clozapine is not only a highly effective antipsychotic, but it can also actually reverse TD. For the first time, it was clear that antipsychotic effects were not irrevocably linked with the risk for TD. Unfortunately, as exciting as clozapine was, it has enough serious side effects of its own to make its widespread use problematic. One of the most concerning is its potential for destroying a person's ability to make blood cells (aplastic anemia). Although this side effect is rare (about 1 to 3 percent), the only way to prevent the potentially fatal consequences is early detection, so patients taking clozapine must have their blood checked every one to two weeks. Why clozapine has such a different profile continues to be of interest to researchers. Like all antipsychotics, it blocks the dopamine receptors, but it also affects receptors of a number of other brain neuroregulators. Somehow, that balance of effects results in the lowered risk for TD.

Once it was clear that TD and drug efficacy were not connected, the search for similar drugs began and resulted in a wave of new drugs, beginning with risperidone in the late 1990s. These "atypical" antipsychotics were greeted with considerable fanfare and a remarkably swift change from the old antipsychotics to the new ones ensued.

As experience with these newer antipsychotics has grown, we are again reminded that no drugs are perfect. Indeed, the risk of TD is far lower with these newer drugs, although it is probably not zero. Also, these new classes of drugs come with their own side effects. The effects of the atypical antipsychotics on appetite and certain aspects of body metabolism are particularly remarkable. Many patients who take these new drugs describe an intense need to eat, like a void in their stomach they must fill. Astonishing gains in weight sometimes result. A few years ago, I had a patient who had been placed on several medications when he was only three

---

REASONS FOR USING ANTIPSYCHOTICS IN CHILDREN AND ADOLESCENTS

DISORDERS

> Psychosis (schizophrenia, mania, psychotic depression, other psychoses)
> Tourette's disorder and other severe motor tic disorders*
> Severe ADHD unresponsive to other treatments

SEVERE BEHAVIORS

> Uncontrollable agitation, aggression, or rage
> Self-injurious behaviors
> Extreme impulsivity
> Perseverative behaviors (continuing the same behavior far beyond reasonable limits)
> Stereotypies (repetitive movements such as hand flapping)
> Labile mood usually leading to tantrums or rages

*Only some antipsychotics are effective for tics; see table on antipsychotics used in children and adolescents.

and a half because of severe behavioral outbursts. When I met him at age five, he had been on risperidone and then olanzapine for about nine months. During that time, he had doubled his body weight, going from a normal-weight young boy to a grossly obese one who could barely walk down a hallway. Such extreme weight gain is not normal, but increases of ten or fifteen pounds over the first few months are not at all uncommon, even with careful monitoring of dietary habits.

In 2000, clinicians began to report that patients on atypical antipsychotics were not only gaining weight, but were also showing an unexpectedly high risk for developing type-2 (sometimes called adult-onset) diabetes and marked elevations in blood cholesterol and other lipids. It is possible that these changes are a result of drug-induced obesity, but some research suggests that this is only part of the problem.

Thus, there are now new drugs that have distinct and clear advantages over the older drugs but also have major drawbacks, including the need for regular blood tests to monitor for metabolic changes, something that was not needed with the older drugs. Parents and physicians are left to work together to decide between a substantive risk of TD versus an even larger likelihood of obesity and possible life-endangering development of diabetes and hypercholesterolemia. With children,

these decisions are even more difficult because of the lack of systematic research with this age group. Of the atypical antipsychotics, to date only risperidone has been subjected to any amount of systematic research in children, and this research was only in the context of autism.

Dosage

Adjusting the dosage of antipsychotic medications might be considered more of an art than a science, and must be accomplished through a bit of trial and error. The potential range of effective dosages is quite large, and the actual dose needed will vary based on the age and size of the patient, the disorder or symptom being treated, and the side effects experienced. Sometimes several medications must be tried to find the right one. Like many of the other medications discussed, they take time to get into the system, so it also takes time to see if there are negative side effects.

Perhaps my strongest rule, especially for this class of medications, is an adage one of my mentors taught me when I first started prescribing medications for children: "Start low, go slow." I typically begin with a dose well below what I think a child needs, because some patients respond even to very low doses. Then I raise the dose slowly, especially when the problems are severe. This is not due to a lack of empathy for the pain patients and parents are experiencing, but rather it is the result of what happens when I've rushed into increased doses early on. For example, one higher-functioning adolescent with autism was agitated much of the time, and we agreed on a trial of haloperidol. I started him on 1 mg twice a day, which, based on my work with adults, seemed a reasonable dose for someone his age. After his second dose on the first day, he had such severe muscle spasms and rigidity that he was unable to walk; I promptly gave him the medication used to treat that side effect, only to have him react to that by being completely unable to urinate. Eventually, he responded nicely to 0.25 mg twice a day.

As the underlying problem changes, dose needs may vary. Parents often become adept at reading their child and knowing what times of the year or types of challenges may cause more behavioral problems that demand more medications. This needs to be done in consultation with the prescribing doctor but can lead to a far more satisfactory overall response using lower doses of medication.

Most antipsychotic medications can be given just once a day, although some families prefer to give them more often. Younger children tend to be fast metabolizers, so multiple doses a day may help smooth out the benefits. Also, side effects are often worst when the medicine levels are highest in the bloodstream. Spreading out the dose or giving it all at bedtime can help to avoid some side effects.

Antipsychotics are not addictive. Although sedation can decrease over time, most of the benefits continue indefinitely. If a child needs higher doses, it usually is because of metabolic changes that occur with puberty or because of growth during development. This class of medications has little to no abuse potential and is not something other children are likely to take from your child, at least not more than once.

Side Effects

Side effects are different for everyone, and you should immediately bring any negative change in function or behavior to the attention of the doctor. If you're not sure that it's a side effect, ask—there's no need for you to hold back your concern. Although the doctor should have gone over common side effects in advance, unusual ones happen plenty of times too.

Common side effects of antipsychotic medications include drowsiness, weight gain, loss of menstrual cycles in women, dizziness when standing up (caused by a drop in blood pressure), drooling, dry mouth, and blurred vision. One common set of side effects especially common with high-potency typical antipsychotics can be stiffness, trembling, and cramping of voluntary muscles. This cramping, called dystonia, can be especially anxiety-producing and even painful. It can affect a wide range of muscles including the eyes, neck, arms, and legs. These side effects are often called extrapyramidal reactions (EPRs) or Parkinsonian side effects, because they resemble symptoms that occur in Parkinson's disease, a disorder resulting from destruction of dopamine neurons in a specific part of the brain. In general, more potent antipsychotics are more likely to produce EPRs. With antipsychotics that have a high likelihood of producing EPRs, such as haloperidol and higher doses of risperidone, physicians will often recommend a second medication, called an anticholinergic, to prevent the side effect.

As mentioned earlier, about 15 to 20 percent of people who are on typical antipsychotics for a long time develop tardive dyskinesia. TD is a rhythmic, largely involuntary movement of some part of the body, frequently the mouth, tongue, fingers, or toes. It may start with lip smacking and tongue rolling and may progress to other facial movements including eye blinks and grimacing. Higher doses of typical antipsychotics actually mask TD symptoms but also worsen their severity over time. Lowering or stopping the drug initially results in a prompt worsening of symptoms, followed usually by slow improvement. Roughly half of those who develop TD will eventually have a complete remission of symptoms if the antipsychotic is discontinued, but they also lose the benefits the drug was providing.

An infrequent but severe reaction to antipsychotic medications is called neuroleptic malignant syndrome. This is a medical emergency, with key symptoms including severe muscle tightness, confusion, sweating, fever, and unstable blood pressure and pulse. If your child develops any of these symptoms, immediately go to the emergency room.

The Bottom Line

Antipsychotics are an important component of the pharmacological arsenal for child and adolescent psychiatrists, who are usually the most experienced with and the most skilled in prescribing these medications for young patients. Reality has tempered hopes from a few years ago that the atypical antipsychotics would be markedly safer than the older ones, but the available medications in this class offer a reasonable array of options. Just keep in mind that, even when they work optimally, they do not cure the underlying problem; however, they may well make life notably better for all concerned.

Mood Stabilizers

Some people find the term "mood stabilizer" offensive or negative, arguing that it is reminiscent of the days of "chemical straitjackets," when patients were so heavily medicated that they were unable to feel either the highs or lows of life. I would share their attitude if this were the intent or reality of what mood stabilizers do. However, just as antidepressants cannot prevent one from having depressed thoughts, mood stabilizers cannot restrict the moods of those who take them to a narrow band of acceptable emotions. What they can do, when they work properly, is tame the raging extremes of emotions that can be so devastating for individuals with bipolar, disruptive, or explosive mood disorders.

Most people have violent thoughts at some point, but they know not to act on them. Children who have trouble controlling these impulses may suffer from ADHD, conduct disorder, psychosis, mood disorder, intermittent explosive disorder, adjustment disorder, personality disorders, mental retardation, or delirium. Mood stabilizers, which include lithium and various anticonvulsants, are used when it becomes necessary to control explosive behavioral and emotional swings, aggressiveness, or agitation. These medications have both antimanic and antidepressant actions.

Persistent agitation itself is a complex behavior with many potential causes, only some of which respond to medication. For example, reactions to an excessively chaotic environment or rage from chronic physical or emotional abuse are unlikely to respond to mood stabilizers. If, however, the behavior seems to occur even in a supportive environment in which external sources of distress are minimal, mood stabilizers may have a role in treatment. These symptoms are quite common in severe forms of ADHD, especially in those children who suffer from other overlapping disorders.

Scott, age seven, had a lifelong history of abrupt mood changes with sustained, furious tantrums, often over trivial frustrations such as having to wait a few minutes before having a snack. During the tantrums, which often occurred daily and could last for twenty to forty minutes each time, Scott would rage verbally and physically, trying to break anything he could grab, even items precious to him. Afterward, he was always immensely and sincerely sorry, calling himself stupid and horrible and saying that maybe everyone would be better off if he were dead. His background revealed no family history of mental illness and his intelligence level was normal, but he was performing badly in school because of his rages there. Not surprisingly, he also had no friends. After considering a variety of options, his parents and I agreed to a trial of valproic acid (Depakote), and Scott was comfortable with the plan. Starting was hard, and he experienced some weight gain and daytime sleepiness. We raised the dose slowly, and gradually Scott and those around him noticed a difference: His tantrums were less frequent, less violent, and shorter.

After about four months on the medication, Scott observed that he might still feel the urge to tantrum but could choose not to, which was extremely exciting for him. A year later, Scott had not experienced a tantrums for three months. We agreed to stop his medication over the summer; however, when we had decreased his daily dose by about 75 percent, Scott

LIVING WITH A CHILD WITH BIPOLAR DISORDER

Glenda was sixteen years old when her family first consulted me. Before age eleven, she was a loving daughter, superb student, and caring friend. Then she went through her "black period," where she lost all interest in friends, family, and school. She became defiant and rebellious, started using a variety of drugs and alcohol, and began getting Ds and Fs in school, which she rarely bothered to attend.

Her parents thought she was coming out of her phase a few months before bringing her to me, when all of a sudden she seemed full of energy, began interacting with others in a much more positive manner, and started to take an interest in school. Unfortunately, she couldn't concentrate or even sit still long enough to do homework. A psychological assessment showed problems with inattention, impulsivity, and hyperactivity, leading to a suggestion that she had ADHD, even though she had none of those problems when younger.

When the family came to see me for a second opinion, I learned that Glenda was only sleeping a few hours a night, complained of "racing thoughts," and was beginning to feel that she had special powers. I diagnosed her with bipolar disorder, and started her on lithium. A few months later, she was back in school full-time, was once more as the all-As student she had once been; in fact, she caught up on three years of backlogged schoolwork in less than a year.

---

had a tantrum. We raised the dose to about half the former amount, and he remained tantrum free for the next several years.

About Mood Stabilizers

The history of mood stabilizers is one that illustrates how serendipity often plays a key role in influencing our discovery of medications useful for those with mental illness. The first medicine used as a mood stabilizer was lithium. Its effects on mood were discovered in 1949 by John Cade, an Australian physician convinced that the key to understanding mania lay in isolating what he believed to be a toxic substance present in the patients' urine. He believed he had found the toxic agent and sought to cleanse manic patients of it with a compound that happened to contain lithium. He observed, first in animals and then in humans, that lithium was sedating and calming. Preliminary trials in humans produced remarkable benefits, as often happens with initial studies, but these encouraging findings were then affirmed with larger, better-controlled studies in Europe. Lithium did not win approval for the treatment of bipolar disorder in the U.S. until 1969. However, despite extensive research, there is still little understanding of how a simple atom can have such a profound effect on mood. However, some evidence suggests it "stabilizes" the neuronal membrane, which some suggest might make brain systems less reactive, and therefore less prone to abrupt changes.

As is true for nearly all medications, lithium is not right for everyone, either because it fails to work or it has unacceptable side effects. As a result, clinicians began to look for drugs with similar benefits during the late 1970s. One logical place to look for an alternative was with the anticonvulsants used to treat seizures, since they also seem to stabilize the neuronal membrane. Sure enough, one such anticonvulsant, carbamazepine (Tegretol) proved beneficial for patients with bipolar disorder. Later, valproic acid (Depakote), another anticonvulsant, was also shown to have good effect. For a time, psychiatrists assumed that every new anticonvulsant would be an effective mood stabilizer, but this is not the case, and it is still uncertain why some work and others do not.

Concurrent to their work with bipolar disorder, psychiatrists were also exploring what other disorders might respond to lithium. Because lithium calms manic patients, who can sometimes be quite aggressive, it was tested on nonmanic individuals with severe aggressive behaviors. Again, research showed notable benefits. Because teenagers with conduct disorder often get into trouble from aggressive outbursts, lithium was also tested in that pop-

MOOD STABILIZERS USED IN CHILDREN AND ADOLESCENTS

Drug	Typical Dose (mg/day)	Doses (per day)
Lithium	300–2400	2
ANTICONVULSANTS		
Carbamazepine (Tegretol)	100–1000	2–3
Valproic acid (Depakote)	125–5000*	2–3
Lamotrigine (Lamictal)**	25–400	1
Oxcarbazepine (Trileptal)	600–2400	2
ATYPICAL (Second-Generation) ANTIPSYCHOTICS		
Aripiprazole (Abilify)	2.5–20	1–2
Olanzapine (Zyprexa)	2.5–20	1–4
Quetiapine (Seroquel)	25–800	1–4
Risperidone (Risperdal)*	0.25–8	1–4
Ziprasidone (Geodon)*	20–160	1–2

*dosage calculated by weight, ranging from 15–60 mg/kg/day

**strong recommendations against usage below age twelve because of serious skin rashes

ulation, with modestly positive results. The drugs carbamazepine and then valproic acid also resemble lithium in their benefits for bipolar disorder, and both these drugs have been tested for, and often are used to treat, aggressive behavior and (to a lesser extent) conduct disorder.

Before lithium became the choice among mood stabilizers, physicians used antipsychotics to treat mania; they are still used for aggressive behaviors. With the huge popularity of the atypical antipsychotics, researchers began looking at their usefulness as mood stabilizers. Although there are some differences in the reaction the atypical antipsychotics produced, the FDA has endorsed them as safe and effective treatments for bipolar disorder in adults. Not surprisingly, studies on aggression and conduct disorder are underway.

Classes of Mood Stabilizers

As summarized in the table discussing mood stabilizers used in children and adolescents, mood stabilizers fall into three categories: Lithium, anticonvulsants, and atypical antipsychotics. The atypical antipsychotics are discussed in detail in Chapter 9. Because the other mood stabilizers are so different from each other, each one will be described separately.

Lithium

Lithium is a highly effective medication with potentially serious side effects. When effective, it can help patients with bipolar disorder avoid the highs and lows of the disorder with little, if any, change in their thinking processes or overall reactions to others. In short, it can make people feel normal.

For those who can recall their periodic charts, you'll remember that lithium is an element, a metal closely related to sodium. It is naturally present (in trace amounts) in the body and may have been an important component in the waters of some health spas popular in the nineteenth and early twentieth centuries. Medicinally, lithium is administered as a salt (usually lithium carbonate), and it looks and even tastes much like table salt

(sodium chloride). In fact, one of the reasons lithium took so long to become available in the U.S. was because physicians in the 1930s used it as a substitute for table salt for patients with high blood pressure or hypertension. They had to stop using it as a salt substitute because some patients would use such large amounts that it became toxic, so physicians were convinced it simply was too dangerous to use as a medication.

The effective range of lithium is relatively narrow: too little, and it fails to help; too much, and it causes severe side effects, even death. Because each body handles lithium differently, the only way to be sure that a person is on the right dose is to draw blood and measure the amount of lithium in it. This is usually done twelve hours after a dose has been taken. Your doctor or the laboratory performing the test will know the appropriate range; but an amount even less than twice a concentration in that range can still be toxic. Slow- or controlled-release lithium is available, and most doctors initially prescribe 300–450 mg once or twice a day. Some patients respond well to a low dose, others need to have the dosage increased until they achieve a therapeutic blood concentration.

Typically, once a patient reaches a desired concentration, the dose needed to keep that concentration in the blood

DISORDERS

    Bipolar disorder

    Conduct disorder

SEVERE BEHAVIORS

    Uncontrollable agitation, aggression, or rage

    Labile mood usually leading to tantrums or rages

remains about the same. However, strenuous exercise with inadequate hydration or physical illness with fever and changes in fluid intake can affect blood concentrations. Early toxicity can mimic flu symptoms, so illness can be an especially difficult time for those on lithium; they may need repeated blood tests to make sure a high lithium concentration is not adding to their symptoms.

Common signs of toxic amounts of lithium include marked tremors, nausea, diarrhea, blurred vision, dizziness (vertigo), confusion, and increased deep-tendon reflexes. With even higher blood concentrations, patients may experience more severe neurological complications and eventually experience seizures, coma, cardiac arrhythmia, permanent neurological damage, and death.

Even at appropriate blood concentrations, lithium commonly produces side effects. Most of these are minor and can be reduced or eliminated by lowering the lithium dose or changing the dosage schedule. The most common short-term side effects are gastrointestinal: Patients may experience symptoms such as nausea, upset stomach, and vomiting. Lithium may also cause substantial weight gain and may worsen acne.

Long-term use of lithium carries the risk of affecting the function of the thyroid gland, producing hypothyroidism in about one-third of patients, and perhaps even more in prepubertal children. Hypothyroidism is a common disorder even without the use of lithium, and medications are available to treat it, although it still requires routine monitoring. More controversial evidence suggests that lithium may adversely affect the kidneys. Everyone shows gradual loss of kidney function with age, but lithium may speed up that process, although probably not at a rate that causes clinical problems. Still, doctors should monitor kidney function periodically.

Complicated as this all may sound—and lithium is a medication that most pediatricians will not and should not prescribe—the benefits from this drug can be so profound that it continues to be an important part of the therapeutic program.

Anticonvulsants

Although anticonvulsants are used widely in children with seizure disorders, there is still little information available about their use as mood stabilizers in young individuals with bipolar disorder or aggressive behaviors. Most of the information about these drugs comes from research done on adults, with results extrapolated for a younger population.

Carbamazepine

Carbamazepine (Tegretol) was the first anticonvulsant shown to function as a mood stabilizer, and it has been used in children for many years, although actual research on its safety and efficacy is sparse. It is structurally related to tricyclic antidepressants, but it is not especially useful as an antidepressant itself. Its use has decreased largely because of the difficulties entailed in using it.

Carbamazepine has the unusual prop-erty of inducing its own metabolism: As the dose is raised, the liver becomes increasingly active in breaking the substance down into an inactive form. As a result, a higher dose can cause a patient to actually have a lower blood concentration. Like with lithium, blood concentrations must be monitored closely, especially at first, and blood should be drawn roughly twelve hours after the last dose. Once an appropriate dose is reached, it is relatively stable over time but still requires monitoring several times a year.

Like lithium, carbamazepine has a fairly narrow "therapeutic window," meaning that the difference between a dose that is too low and one that is too high is relatively small. At higher concentrations, patients experience toxic reactions such as slurred speech, nausea, vomiting, drowsiness, confusion, and nystagmus (rhythmic movement of the eyes side to side). Abrupt discontinuation of the drug can sometimes result in seizures.

Even in the therapeutic range, carbamazepine can produce a variety of side effects ranging from minor to serious. Lesser side effects include nausea, dizziness, double vision (diplopia), and rash. More infrequent but more serious problems include an especially dangerous skin rash called Stevens-Johnson syndrome and bone marrow suppression.

Valproic Acid

Valproic acid (Depakote) has been popular among child and adolescent psychiatrists for the past ten to fifteen years, but its use now seems to be waning. Compared to lithium and carbamazepine, valproic acid is easier to use. There are no problems with metabolism, and there is less need to closely monitor blood concentrations. There have been studies of use in adolescents with bipolar and conduct disorders, but results have not been sufficient to convince the FDA to endorse its use in either condition in patients under eighteen.

When patients first start valproic acid, they often feel lethargic during the day, although this usually improves with time. Overdoses of valproic acid produce drowsiness, weakness, confusion, and decreased coordination. Common side effects at therapeutic doses include gastrointestinal symptoms such as vomiting and diarrhea as well as weight gain, tremors, and hair loss (alopecia). Although not all medical professionals agree that this is a side effect, some feel that long-term use in women may increase their risk for polycystic ovary disease, which may affect child-bearing potential. It is also associated with rare, but potentially fatal, liver toxicity and with Stevens-Johnson syndrome. Valproic acid also interferes directly with folic acid absorption, so supplementation with a vitamin containing folic acid is recommended.

Other Anticonvulsants

Given the complexities of the three best-studied mood stabilizers, it is probably no surprise that the search for more viable alternatives continues. The atypical antipsychotics seemed likely candidates, but the problems surrounding their use make them less appealing than initially thought. Psychiatrists also continue to mine the anticonvulsants for possible additional mood stabilizers. The introduction of each new anticonvulsant inevitably leads to a flurry of case reports and open-label studies suggesting that it may also be beneficial for bipolar disorder. Two medications for which such hopes may be justified are lamotrigine (Lamictal) and oxcarbazepine (Tripleptal). The former carries an FDA endorsement for use in bipolar disorder in adults, and the latter is under investigation in both adolescents and adults. However, lamotrigine has such serious potential for severe skin rash in children under age twelve that its use in younger patients is strongly discouraged. Oxcarbazepine is structurally related to carbamazepine and has the advantage of not inducing its own metabolism, but its benefits as a mood stabilizer remain uncertain.

The Bottom Line

Mood stabilizers are a powerful group of medications that can be of considerable benefit to the right patient. However, their use is complicated enough to be beyond the expertise of most pediatricians. These are intense drugs and should only be used for serious behavior problems that have failed to respond to other alternative approaches. Since few child neurologists are willing to treat children or adolescents with mental disorders, child psychiatrists are the ones most likely to help you decide if one of these medications is right for your child.

Chapter 11

Stimulants and Other ADHD Medications

The first clinical observations of the impact of stimulants on what was then called hyperactivity occurred in the late 1930s, at the dawn of modern psychopharmacology. Stimulants are both the crown jewel and the bane of child psychopharmacology. No medicine available to psychiatrists produces a more rapid and dramatic effect more safely than the proper dose of a stimulant to a patient with ADHD. Again and again, researchers have demonstrated the ability of stimulants to reverse the key symptoms of inattention, hyperactivity, and impulsivity with remarkable precision and relatively minor side effects. I routinely encourage my psychiatry trainees to witness this phenomenon directly by asking a family to bring in their child before he or she receives the usual daily dose. The trainee can experience firsthand the child who tears around the office, impulsively getting into everything but not staying with anything for long because the next unexplored item beckons. After administering the stimulant, the trainee can witness the transformation, which takes no longer than thirty minutes, as that same patient turns into a far more normal child—quieter, more polite, and able to stay on task.

At the same time, stimulants highlight many of the frustrations of child and adolescent psychiatrists and the patients and families with whom they work. They are not effective for everyone; although an 85 percent response rate is excellent for field, it leaves 15 percent who continue to suffer. In addition, although the effects are prompt, they are also transient. It is clear these medications do not change whatever lies at the core of ADHD; rather, they target its manifestations. Also, despite years of innovative research, how stimulants affect the course of this potentially devastating disorder over time is still uncertain. Does early treatment affect later outcome? If so, how?

In addition to these medical issues, there are also political issues surrounding the use of stimulants. Interestingly, the two largest populations that use stimulants are at social extremes. On one side falls the socioeconomically disadvantaged children, often black or Hispanic, who are disruptive in school; and on the other are middle- to upper-class children, often white, whose parents want to ensure they do as well as possible in school. Are stimulants being used as a "chemical straitjacket" or as a questionable performance enhancer? Evidence suggests that, at certain times, the answer to both is yes. And yet, research also plainly shows that many children with severe ADHD who could benefit from these medications never receive them.

Despite these issues, stimulants have proven highly effective for the management of acute ADHD symptoms. Furthermore, starting in the late 1990s, options have expanded not only in the types of formulations available for stimulants but also in nonstimulant alternatives for treating ADHD.

The late 1980s and the 1990s were a time of major attitude shifts concerning the use of stimulants for treating ADHD. Researchers convincingly demonstrated that ADHD could affect adolescents and adults as severely as it does younger children. In addition, conventional wisdom that ADHD was a problem limited to school hours yielded to empirical evidence that it also affects many other aspects of life, including leisure time activities, peer relationships, and home life. A broad consensus among researchers, clinicians, affected families, and patients called for more vigorous identification and treatment of ADHD. This has included both more intense treatment at any time, longer during each day, for more days of the week, and more weeks of the year, but also over time—into adolescence and even adulthood.

Stimulants

The two major classes of stimulants available in the U.S. are amphetamine and methylphenidate (see table on stimulants used in children and adolescents). Since stimulants first entered common use in the 1960s for treating hyperactivity, public attitudes about them have varied widely—from hailing them as miracle drugs to vilifying them as brain poisons. As is so often is the case, the truth lies somewhere in between.

Since 1989, use of stimulants in the U.S. has expanded greatly, especially during the late 1990s. Although evidence suggests this is probably a good thing for children with ADHD, there is little question that it has resulted in problems of diversion and

STIMULANTS USED IN CHILDREN AND ADOLESCENTS

Drug	Typical Dose (mg/day)	Doses (per day)	Expected Duration (hours/dose)
METHYLPHENIDATE			
Concerta	18–72	1	10–12
Focalin	2.5–30	1–3	2.5–4
Focalin XR	5–30	1	10–12
generic	5–60	1–3	2.5–3
Metadate ER	10–60	1	8–10
Metadate CD	10–60	1	8–10
Methylin	10–60	1–3	2.5–3
Methylin ER	10–60	1	8–10
Ritalin	5–60	1–3	2.5–3
Ritalin LA	20–60	1	8–10
AMPHETAMINE			
Adderall	5–40	1–2	3–4
Adderall XR	10–40	1	10–12
Dextrostat	5–30	1–2	3–4
Dexedrine	5–30	1–2	3–4
Dexedrine ER	10–30	1	8–12
generic	5–30	1–2	3–4

misuse. Parents contemplating giving a stimulant to their child must be aware of the controversies that accompany this class of drugs.

Methylphenidate and amphetamine are called stimulants because they activate parts of the brain. Studies in animals and adult subjects show that they have a variety of effects, including increased alertness and energy, decreased tiredness, and improved ability to tend to even dull and repetitive tasks without errors. These effects may be mediated by an increase in dopamine, a neurotransmitter involved in the reward centers of the brain.

Parents often ask why anyone would be silly enough to give a brain stimulant to a child who already has too much energy. This is a valid question, and one that again shows how essential it is to differentiate children from adults. In pre-pubescent children, stimulants enhance attention and focus as they do in adults, but actually tend to reduce physical activity and energy. This is true whether a child has ADHD or not, something not known until the late 1970s. Before that, clinicians mistakenly believed that stim-ulants were a good diagnostic tool for ADHD: If the child grew less active and more attentive, he must have ADHD. Occasionally, you may still find physi-cians who adhere to this antiquated belief, but it is simply not true. Diagnosis of ADHD takes a lot more than observing a child respond to a medication.

Benefits and Drawbacks

While every drug has some side effects, **stimulants have several advantages:**

- They have a long history of use in children. Although there is still much to learn, clinicians have been using methylphenidate and amphetamine regularly in children and young adoles-cents since the 1960s, and these drugs have been studied more extensively than any other psychoactive drug prescribed for children. Studies have repeatedly shown them to be safe and effective for reducing ADHD symptoms.
- Stimulants start and stop working quickly. The effects of immediate-release formulations begin within twenty to thirty minutes and are essen-tially out of the body after a few hours. Any behavioral effects are gone by the next day.
- Stimulants work for a remarkably high percentage of patients. Research suggests that between 85 to 90 percent of children with combined-type ADHD will respond to one of the available medications.
- The benefits persist over time for the key symptoms of ADHD in properly diagnosed individuals. Patients do not grow tolerant to the stimulant effects and need higher and higher doses, as occurs in stimulant abuse.

Despite this, knowledge about stimu-lants is still incomplete. For example, most studies to date have focused on school-aged boys, and only a few have studied medication effects beyond a few weeks. Worse, essentially nothing is known about the long-term benefits and problems of stimulant treatment for ADHD and how early treatment may affect adolescence and adulthood.

Given what is known, the continuing level of public wariness about stimulants is impressive. Early in 2005, the Canadian government abruptly withdrew Adderall XR from the market after analyzing reports of twenty deaths worldwide in children and adults taking this drug, often in combination with several others. Deaths of any sort are cause for concern, and there is clear evidence that people who abuse stimulants such as methamphetamine or cocaine put themselves at risk for heart problems and sudden death. But were these deaths the fault of Adderall? Interestingly, the U.S. FDA examined the same data in 2004 and concluded that Adderall was not a concern. In late 2005, after widespread protests from parents whose children had been deprived of a beneficial medication and upon further careful review of the data, Canada reversed its decision and reinstated Adderall XR.

In early 2006, the U.S. FDA revisited the possibility of sudden death associated with the use of stimulants, both methylphenidate and amphetamine. A panel of cardiovascular experts reviewed a small number of reported deaths (fewer than fifty in the past ten years) thought to have occurred as a direct or indirect result of a therapeutic dose of a stimulant. The panel recommended a "black-box warning"— the FDA's mechanism for emphasizing especially worrisome side effects—arguing that patients and parents needed to know. Final action has yet to be taken by the FDA.

Dosage and Frequency

How should you and your prescribing doctor choose which stimulant is right for your child? In essence, it really doesn't matter all that much. No reliable methods exist yet for pairing a specific type of stimulant medication to a particular patient, and general response rates are so high that usually the first choice has an excellent chance of success. As a result, many physicians have become comfortable with one particular type or formulation of stimulant and will probably prescribe that one for your child. Even so, if you have prior positive or negative experiences with a particular type of stimulant, let the physician know, so your concern can be part of the decision-making process.

I usually begin by talking with the family about where the problems are and what prior experiences they have had. We will go through a routine weekday from morning to bedtime, talking about what goes smoothly and what does not from both the child's and parents' point of view. Input from teachers, after-school programs, sports coaches, and others involved in the child's life is also important. I also ask about prior medication use, whether the child knows how to swallow pills, and what side effects would be unacceptable. Once the bigger picture is established, we can decide where to start.

I typically recommend that parents give the first dose of a stimulant on a weekend or during a holiday, so they can see for themselves what kinds of changes do and do not occur with their child. When I first started in child psychiatry, I was stunned to learn that some parents had their child on stimulants for years but had literally never seen any of the effects. Children would receive a dose just as they headed out the door for school and then a second dose later in the morning. It would have worn off by the time they got home, and they didn't take medication on the weekend. I believe it's essential for parents to know how their child is doing. If there is a

A BIG DIFFERENCE

Jan, a bright ten-year-old, had notable problems with inattention and class participation, but was doing well academically. Middle school was especially problematic for her because she had so many different classes and teachers. Her parents arranged for her to go to an after-school program to help her get through her homework, and on evenings and weekends she seemed fine. Jan wanted to try medication because she was sure she could do better academically if she could pay better attention to her teachers. She was of normal weight but a picky eater, and had never learned to swallow pills. Sleep had never been a problem. We decided to try Ritalin LA, and two of her teachers agreed to fill out a brief checklist three times a week to assess her key issues in the classroom. In addition, her parents agreed to monitor and record how the medication affected her appetite and sleep. We decided not to teach Jan how to swallow pills right then, since we could sprinkle the medication over her cereal.

On Saturday, a first dose of 10 mg of Ritalin LA showed no change, which actually comforted both Jan and her parents, all of whom had worried that she might lose her personality. A week of 10 mg of Ritalin LA at school showed no real change and no side effects. Increasing the dose to 20 mg a day the next week, however, led to dramatic increases in class participation and improved focus. The after-school tutor reported that Jan whizzed through her homework without nearly as much prompting. Her parents noted no side effects, except that Jan no longer wanted to eat lunch. A trial of 30 mg had no clear additional benefits at school but resulted in clear appetite suppression at both lunch and supper, with a return of appetite just before bedtime. Also, Jan found it harder to get to sleep, taking up to forty-five minutes longer to get to sleep each night. We agreed to return to 20 mg a day and decided that she would take medication only on school days.

problem, they'll know, and we can work at fixing it. If there isn't one, they'll feel better about their child's medication.

Beyond the medication, we will also pick several key target symptoms to track, as well as possible side effects. I try to keep the list short, no more than four to six symptoms and a comparable number of side effects. I usually encourage parents to make up their own sheet of benefits and drawbacks.

After all this has been done, I then start the child on a low dose of the agreed-upon medication and ask the parents to fill out their rating sheet several times each week. When possible, getting teacher input is very helpful. Usually, four to seven days is plenty of time to see if the child is doing well at the initial dose—it is enough time to make sure a bad or good day isn't mistaken for a negative or positive response, and stimulants do not take much time to start working. If there are no benefits and no side effects, the dose is increased. If side effects do emerge, I tend to wait a few days to see if they improve, which they usually do. Once clear benefits begin to appear, the focus shifts to balancing increasing improvement with worsening side effects. The response to these medications is pretty consistent as dosages increase. If the same benefits still occur after two increases, additional increases are unlikely to produce any more; however, side effects will eventually begin to appear with higher dosages.

Fine Tuning

It is not always easy to find the right medication, proper dosage, and the right time

---

DIFFERENCES AMONG METHYLPHENIDATE PREPARATIONS

Drug	Form	Release Pattern
Concerta*	insoluble capsule	28% IR, then ascending curve
Focalin XR**	capsule with beads	50% IR, 50% at 4 hours
Metadate CD**	capsule with beads	steady release
Metadate ER*	wax matrix tablet	30% IR, 70% at 4 hours
Ritalin LA**	capsule with beads	50% IR, 50% at 4 hours

*must remain intact to work properly
**sustained release is property of beads; capsules can be opened and sprinkled over food

to adjust it. **Here are a few of the problems that can occur as medication is being fine-tuned for your child:**

- Quitting before reaching an adequate dose. This can cause you to think that the medication is a failure, when it really wasn't given a proper chance.
- Not choosing a medication that covers the key times of the day.
- Not letting the doctor know about side effects, or reluctance to insist that side effects be addressed. It is not unusual to feel intimidated or rushed by medical professionals, but their intention is to help your child and your family. If the medication has side effects that are unpleasant for you or for the child, let the physician know.
- Failing to monitor changes that may affect a child's medication needs, including body weight, pubertal status, and school obligations.
- Assuming that a child who is doing well no longer needs the medicine.
- Choosing the wrong time to stop medication. Periods of transition are challenging for anybody, so if you are going to experiment with taking a child off a medication, work with your doctor so it can happen at a time when the child is in a stable environment; for example, a couple of weeks into summer vacation instead of when school first lets out.

Side Effects

Although stimulants are generally well-tolerated, they do have potential side effects that can, at times, interfere with their efficacy and may require switching to a different type of medication. My involvement in the Multimodal Treatment Study of Children with ADHD (MTA) has been an especially rich opportunity to monitor the side effects of methylphenidate over time, since I have had the opportunity to follow a group of children with combined-type ADHD from entry (ages seven to nine) to midadolescence (ages thirteen to fifteen).

Appetite and Weight

Appetite suppression and resulting effects on weight can be a serious side effect. The effect is dose-dependent, with more than one-third of patients on doses of 50 mg a day or higher complaining of significant appetite suppression. Typically, the effect is immediate, subsiding as the amount in the body decreases. Many find that the effect diminishes over time, even on the same dose. Loss of appetite is not universal, but few patients seem to experience an increase in appetite. Usually, appetite suppression is greatest when the blood concentrations are at their highest. The most common missed meal is lunch, with lesser problems at dinner. Appetite usually returns sometime during the evening, though for some patients it may not do so until bedtime.

Decreased consumption of food leads to weight loss or failure to gain weight at expected rates. This effect can continue for months to years, but data from the MTA suggests that the effect is greatest during the first year or two. After fourteen and twenty-four months, the difference between those consistently on medication and those never on medication was ten to twelve pounds, with less than a four-pound difference by six years.

Parents can help counteract this side effect by making it easy for children to eat when they are hungry. Thus, a good breakfast before medication effects start is key. Usually, appetite returns by dinnertime; if it does not, a healthy before-bedtime snack can be of great help. Medication-free holidays on weekends, school vacations, and during the summer also can be helpful—assuming the child's behavior makes that feasible.

Height

Whether or not the sustained use of a stimulant has an impact on height remains controversial. Over the past two decades, scientific evidence has been unclear and has variously suggested significant effects, no effects, and reversible effects. The MTA and several other studies now seem to indicate that, on average,

children taking stimulants grow more slowly than those not taking stimulants. A comparison of growth after two years in the MTA study showed that children with ADHD who never received medications were actually growing faster than children without ADHD. However, those who took a stimulant throughout the two years grew at a slower rate than those who did not have the disorder. The result was a one-inch difference in height between the medicated and nonmedicated groups; however, the difference at six years was about the same, meaning that the loss was not cumulative.

It is important for parents to monitor their child's growth, and pediatricians have growth charts to make it easier. If the child shows a serious reduction in growth rate, consider trying a different type of stimulant or a nonstimulant treatment. Research results still are unclear whether drug holidays might help, but they may.

Insomnia

Insomnia is a common side effect of stimulants, although 15 percent of individuals, with or without ADHD, actually seem to sleep better with stimulants. Severity of insomnia is dose-related and is typically reduced over time. Still, the MTA showed that, on average, use of stimulants led to a thirty-minute delay of sleep onset, at least

FINDING THE RIGHT BALANCE

Manuel, age seven, had classic combined-type ADHD. He had been hyperactive from birth, had been asked to leave several preschools because of impulsive aggressive behavior, and had barely made it through kindergarten, which he'd started a year late. First grade began on a slightly better note, but the teacher finally called his parents in for a conference because he was not fitting in. Manuel's parents spoke to his pediatrician, who prescribed 5 mg of immediate-release Ritalin, which did nothing, so his parents stopped giving it to Manuel after a few days and did not return to the pediatrician. They finally came to see me in the spring, after another urgent plea from the teacher, who suggested Manuel might need to repeat the first grade.

My assessment affirmed the diagnosis of combined-type ADHD. It also seemed clear that Manuel's problems with math and English were consistent with a learning disorder. Manuel's parents also reported feeling completely ineffective with him. His father worked long hours, and his mother was at home full-time taking care of Manuel and his four-year-old sister. They admitted that his problems weren't limited to school. He was so disruptive at church that he could only go to his Sunday school class if one of his parents went with him. They tried to get Manuel into soccer, which he loved, but he was too easily distracted.

We discussed their prior experience with medication and agreed to try again. We started Manuel on Concerta, because of it has a longer period of efficacy. At a dosage of 18 mg, Manuel showed no benefits or side effects. At 36 mg, parents and teachers both thought he improved mildly, but he had some problems getting to sleep. At 54 mg, he was slightly less active and less impulsive, but his problems with sleep worsened, and his appetite seriously decreased. In addition, he was distinctly more irritable, especially late in the day.

We agreed that the side effects outweighed the benefits, and switched to Adderall XR because it has a similar efficacy period. Manuel started on 20 mg, a little less than the equivalent amount of Concerta. His parents noticed an immediate difference—Manuel had comparable or better benefits but without the irritability and sleeping problems. An increase a week later to 30 mg showed additional benefits but a return of the sleep problem. We decreased the dose to 25 mg each morning, which worked well for him. The school reassessed Manuel for learning problems and concurred that he had delays, which they addressed with a resource class. To everyone's pleasure, his parents were able to get him back into soccer, which he enjoyed much more now that he could pay attention. In addition, his parents took a class that helped them better cope with his impulsivity and disorganization at home, which improved their self-esteem and their relationship with both children.

during the first weeks.

There are perfectly reasonable strategies for dealing with insomnia, including a lower dose, a different stimulant, or a shorter-acting version of the same stimulant. Also important are matters of sleep hygiene; that is, making sure the child is in an environment and has nighttime habits that encourage sleep. Long-term use of a second medication to aid sleep is not uncommon, but no good research exists about either the safety of this practice or the quality of the drug-induced sleep.

Rebound

Rebound is a poorly understood effect of stimulants. For some children, negative behaviors return to off-drug levels as their medication wears off, and they may actually grow worse for a time that may last up to several hours. It is most often seen in children taking short-acting forms of the stimulants. The effect is not clearly dose-related and may or may not diminish with time. Long-acting formulations seem to help diminish rebound, as may adding a smaller dose of an immediate-acting form thirty to sixty minutes before rebound occurs. Trying a different stimulant also may work.

Tics

Motor and vocal tics are common in most young boys. In addition, Tourette disorder, a specific form of tic disorder characterized by both motor and vocal tics, often occurs with symptoms of ADHD. Stimulants may worsen the severity of tics already present and uncover tics in people at risk for having them. The long-term effect of stimulants on tics is less clear. The best available evidence now suggests that a worsening of tics when starting a stimulant does not lead to long-term negative outcomes; in fact, some research suggests that stimulants may actually decrease tic severity in the long term. Still, parents and physicians are understandably reluctant to give a medication that makes tics more severe.

Depending on the child's need and the severity of the tics, parents may want to consider switching to a different stimulant, trying a nonstimulant medication, or continuing use of a stimulant for ADHD while adding another medication to suppress the tics. Each approach has its proponents. If tics persist, it is important to consult with an expert on ADHD and tic disorders.

Cognitive Blunting

While a stimulant's "zombie effect" is familiar to many parents, it has been poorly studied. Cognitive blunting is best defined as a change in mental functioning that results in an apparent slowing of thinking and subdued responses to events.

In the MTA, 25 percent of children on stimulants experienced cognitive blunting. The effect was dose-dependent but could occur even at the lowest dose. It did not always lessen with time.

Approaches to dealing with cognitive blunting include decreasing the dose, as long as it still provides adequate benefits. Sometimes, after several weeks or months, an increased dose will not result in a return of this side effect. Switching to a different stimulant can also work. Otherwise, a nonstimulant medication for ADHD may be the best approach.

Irritability

Parents often describe children on stimulants as being more irritable and edgy. Although this certainly can be true, a surprising finding from the MTA might help prove otherwise. At the beginning of the study, the dose of Ritalin was changed daily for a month without anyone knowing what the daily dose was. Dosages ranged from a placebo (a sugar pill) to as much as 50 mg a day, with two intermediate amounts. Fascinatingly, the highest reports of irritability were in subjects receiving the placebo; less irritability was

NONSTIMULANTS COMMONLY USED FOR ADHD IN CHILDREN AND ADOLESCENTS

Drug	Typical Dose (mg/day)	Doses (per day)	Maximum Dose (per day)
ANTIDEPRESSANTS			
Atomoxetine (Strattera)	10–80	1–2	1.5 mg/kg
Bupropion (Wellbutrin)*	75–450	1–2	450 mg
Imipramine (Tofranil)*	25–300	1–2	3.5 mg/kg
Nortryptline (Pamelor)*	10–150	1–2	3 mg/kg
Venlafaxine (Effexor)*	25–300	1–2	3 mg/kg
OTHER DRUG CLASSES			
Clonidine (Catapres)*	0.05–0.6	1–4	0.8 mg
Guanfacine (Tenex)*	2.5–4	1–2	6 mg
Modafinil (Provigil)*	100–400	1	400 mg

*not FDA-endorsed for treating ADHD

evident as the stimulant dose increased. For this reason, parents should monitor to see if irritability appears as the stimulant is building up, wearing off, or is worst when the stimulant is in full effect.

Irritability often seems to lessen with time. If it does not, trying a different type of stimulant or even a different preparation of the same stimulant may help.

Nonstimulant Medications

Although stimulants work for 80 to 85 percent of those with ADHD, there has been a long-standing interest in other classes of medications that might also be beneficial. Such medications are used in a relative minority of cases, but they can be viable alternatives either for severe cases of ADHD or those for which stimulants otherwise prove unsatisfactory.

In the early 1980s, I first became interested in ADHD because of observations that antidepressants such as imipramine (Tofranil) were effective in treating the disorder. The hypothesis that ADHD is a variant of depression has proven false, but the observations that certain antidepressants can help treat the disorder have held up. These observations have been limited to small research studies and anecdotal clinical observation, with one notable exception. Bupropion (Wellbutrin), which is thought to work by increasing dopamine activity and is used to treat depression, has long been reported to have mild benefits for ADHD, especially for patients with the mainly inattentive subtype.

In 2002, the FDA endorsed a new medication, atomoxetine (Strattera), specifically for ADHD. Atomoxetine is not a stimulant; instead, it increases brain norepinephrine activity, as do several other antidepressants. The endorsement of atomoxetine for ADHD was striking for many reasons, not only because it was the first drug in the modern era to come to market specifically for a childhood mental disorder. The drug company also established its safety and efficacy for adolescents and adults with ADHD.

Atomoxetine works differently from stimulants, requiring several weeks of daily usage before its benefits are apparent and often showing increasing benefit even months later. It must be taken daily, and "holidays" are neither feasible nor desirable. The actual mechanism by which atomoxetine works is poorly understood. The medication's big advantage is that it works more smoothly than stimulants, not only throughout the day and evening but also into the next morning. If morning routines are a major problem for a child, this medication may be worth considering.

The side effects of atomoxetine also differ from those of stimulants. It tends to be too sedating, sometimes causing daytime lethargy. Most common, however, are problems with nausea and vomiting. These problems decrease somewhat with twice-daily dosing and if taken with a meal. Like stimulants, when atomoxetine works, the benefits last over time, without having to increase the dose except to accommodate changes in weight.

Another class of medications of interest for treating ADHD is the alpha-adrenergic agonists. Two medications in this class, clonidine (Catapres) and guanfacine (Tenex), have been under investigation since the late 1980s for their effects on ADHD. Both are mainly used for treating high blood pressure and work by acting directly on certain norepinephrine receptors. Researchers, interested in the possible role of norepineprhine in Tourette's disorder, found that these medications not only reduced tics but also improved measures of attention, impulsivity, and hyperactivity. Subsequent research showed similar benefits with children who had ADHD without tics. Clonidine is extremely sedating, which has limited its use; however, it and guanfacine are used for patients with ADHD who do not tolerate stimulants, or antidepressants such as atomoxetine.

. . . .
Drug Abuse
. . . .

One-third of all drug abuse today is prescription drug abuse, according to the Substance Abuse and Mental Health Services Administration (SAMHSA). In a 2003 Partnership for a Drug-Free America teen study, painkillers were found to be the most common pharmaceuticals abused by teenagers, especially in the younger age groups; stimulant abuse was more common among older teenagers and college students.

Stimulant abuse may start out innocently. The pace of teenagers' lives can be very daunting, and many feel so pressured by school and extracurricular activities that it is not surprising that they may be attracted to a drug that promises to keep them awake to finish their homework. Suppressed appetite may also be a benefit for many concerned about their weight. It's easy to see why they might slip into recurrent stimulant use and then abuse, especially if a mood elevation accompanies the medication. Most children do not experience a sense of elation, and the effects of stimulants on ADHD symptoms do not show evidence of tolerance—patients with ADHD don't need higher and higher doses to maintain the benefits. However, abuse of and addiction to stimulants can occur if the dose is increased enough and especially if method of delivery is improved (i.e., ground up and snorted or dissolved and injected). Unfortunately, there are numerous Web sites that outline how best to abuse these drugs, so it is easy for children to acquire the necessary knowledge. Even more importantly, adolescents with ADHD who are otherwise friendless may find the temptation of bartering their medication for "friends" irresistible.

For the most part, the teenagers who end up in the emergency room for stimulant abuse are not the ones who have prescriptions for the medicines. And, while some stimulants are sold by teenagers who have prescriptions, the recent growth of Web sites selling pharmaceutical drugs has resulted in a higher proportion of children getting their hands on these medications without a prescription. On the black market, stimulants sell for about $3 to $10 per pill.

In general, this issue, like so much of parenting, is a matter of paying attention to changes your child experiences and not assuming, "It can't happen to my child." If in doubt, ask. If the answer makes no sense, keep asking. If you're at all uncertain, make sure to include the doctor in the discussion.

The Bottom Line

Stimulants and other medications known to be effective for ADHD can be of great help in treating this potentially disabling disorder. If you have a young child just starting medication for ADHD, he or she may need treatment for many years, perhaps for life. As with all medications, it is important not to treat this causally. As parents and as physicians, it is too easy to get into the habit of assuming that everything is fine once a helpful medication is found, and simply continue doing what has worked before. It is imperative to reassess the situation with your prescribing doctor every few years to ensure that other needed services are in place, that the medication continues to work as it should, and that new side effects or other problems, such as drug diversion or abuse, are not occurring. This discussion with your doctor can also be an excellent opportunity to review changes in the field and learn about new options and emerging findings from a range of studies.

One of the most distressing aspects of ADHD is its persistence. It is easy to forget how devastating the disorder can be when a child is doing well or to allow old problems to sneak back into family life over months and years. The main focus should always be to help protect the child from the inattention, impulsivity, and resulting issues that are central to this disorder.

Chapter 12

Antianxiety Drugs and Sleeping Pills

Just as the name indicates, antianxiety medications decrease the degree to which people perceive themselves to be anxious, especially in stressful situations. These medications can also reduce the level of general anxiety, causing a person to mellow. Ideally, these drugs do so without otherwise affecting alertness or other cognitive functions. Sometimes called minor tranquilizers (as opposed to the antipsychotics, or major tranquilizers), antianxiety agents generally work best as a brief treatment; for example, when someone has a panic attack or must face a highly stressful situation or event such as a medical or dental procedure.

Long-term use of antianxiety drugs is not recommended because of side effects (impaired alertness, sedation, poor interaction with other drugs), potential for addiction, and problems with withdrawal. In addition, the body can learn to tolerate these medications, so if they are taken for a prolonged period, a patient may need higher and higher doses to achieve the same effect.

Also, the benzodiazepines, one of the classes of antianxiety medications, have effects similar to those of alcohol. Taking the two together has additive effects, potentially impairing judgment and certainly motor coordination and response speeds. Particular caution must be used with adolescents, who may be experimenting with illegal use of alcohol.

Mellow Rats

The first effective antianxiety agent was discovered in the late 1940s when researchers were using rats to test the toxicity of a compound they hoped would be an antibiotic. As the project progressed, the scientists began to notice that the rats given the compound showed significant muscle relaxation and calming without notable sedation. Based on this finding, scientists spent an additional five years modifying the compound to enhance its antianxiety effects. This work eventually led to the discovery of meprobamate, the first medication marketed for anxiety reduction. It and other barbiturates, such as phenobarbital, proved to be addicting and toxic and have largely fallen out of favor. They are still used as street drugs with such names as "barbs," "ludes" (short for Quaalude, one of the more popular members of this class), and "downers."

Discovery of benzodiazepines such as diazepam (Valium) is in some ways even more striking. The first benzodiazapine was synthesized by accident as part of a project that resulted in the production of forty compounds, thirty-nine of which proved to have no significant biological effects. The last compound was shelved, untested, for several years. Chemists were about to discard it but decided to study it before doing so, leading to the discovery of chlordiazepoxide (Librium) and the beginning of the class of compounds that are still safe and potent antianxiety drugs.

But how can these medications help your child feel better? Unfortunately, antianxiety agents are not especially useful for long-term control of anxious symptoms in children. Addiction potential and the need to continually to increase the dosage for consistent effect make it difficult to use these medications for anything but an occasional temporary solution. The benzodiazepines also have a tendency to cause disinhibition (see below), especially in younger patients. Nonetheless, if your child has a chronic problem with anxiety, you should know what is available to help. Since some benzodiazpines were also among the first effective sleeping pills, this chapter will also discuss medications used to help children with serious sleep disturbances.

Types of Antianxiety Medications

Medications used specifically for anxiety include the following:

- **Benzodiazepines**. These are rarely used with prepubertal patients, because of a phenomenon called behavioral disinhibition. A child, or anyone, with behavioral disinhibition can become disoriented, easily angered, and combative. Why children respond in this way is unclear, but the reaction is common enough to discourage routine use of benzodiazepines in this age group.
- **Beta-blockers**. Medications called beta-adrenergic antagonists, mainly used for controlling high blood pressure, are also quite effective at controlling anxiety. The connection was made that controlling the symptoms might lessen the anxiety. Beta-blockers work by controlling the autonomic response of "fight or flight" characterized by

sweaty palms, rapid breathing, pounding heart, and churning stomach. For example, someone fearful of public speaking can take a beta-blocker a few hours before the presentation and go to the podium with dry hands, slowed heartbeat and respirations, and a calm stomach. Many professional musicians and actors use these medications to help them perform.

ANTIANXIETY AGENTS USED IN CHILDREN AND ADOLESCENTS

Drug	Typical Dose (mg/day)	Doses (per day)
BENZODIAZAPINES		
alprazolam (Xanax)*	0.5–4	1–4
chlordiazepoxide (Librium)*	10–100	1–4
clonazapam (Klonopin)*	0.5–6	1–4
diazepam (Valium)*	5–40	1–4
lorazepam (Ativan)*	2.5–100	1–4
ANTIHISTAMINES		
diphenhydramine (Benadryl)	25–200	1–4
hydroxyzine (Vistaril)*	10–250	1–4
BETA-ADRENERGIC ANTAGONISTS		
atenolol (Tenormin)*	5–100	1–2
propranolol (Inderal)*	10–240	1–4
buspirone (BuSpar)*	20–90	2–3
NON-BENZODIAZPINE SLEEPING PILLS		
eszopiclone (Lunesta)*	1–3	1
melatonin	0.5–1	1
zaleplon (Sonata)*	5–10	1
zolpidem (Ambien)*	5–10	1

*few to no studies of safety and efficacy in children

- **Buspirone (BuSpar)** This medication came onto the market about twenty years ago, and it carries an FDA endorsement for adults for treatment of generalized anxiety disorder (GAD). It works differently than benzodiazepines and has some unique properties, including a remarkable dearth of side effects— so few that I once had an adult patient ask if I'd just given him a placebo. One drawback is that it takes several weeks to be effective. Another is that its effects are relatively subtle and mild, so it isn't potent enough for the more serious levels of agitation and distress. It has not been extensively studied in children or adolescents, but in my experience it can sometimes lead to a gradual but significant reduction in anxiety. Interestingly, it is used much more commonly as an adjunct to antidepressants, especially SSRIs, because it helps to reduce the anxiety and restlessness that SSRIs can sometimes cause.

What Doctors Use for Anxious Children

If these antianxiety medications are unlikely to be used on children, **what do physicians use to treat anxiety?**

- **Antihistamines**. For sedation or a relatively fast-acting calming medication, physicians frequently rely on antihistamines such as diphenhydramine (Benadryl), which is available without a prescription and widely used for treating seasonal allergies. These drugs have been used for many years to temporarily reduce anxiety and behavioral disruptions. They seem unlikely to cause behavioral disinhibition, but their efficacy diminishes over time, if they are used too frequently and for too long.
- **SSRIs and other antidepressants**. Antidepressants have been shown to be effective for sustained control of severe anxiety. However, at least in adolescents, benzodiazepines are often an effective adjunct to the antidepressants that help with surges of anxiety or panic attacks.

How They Work

Different classes of antianxiety agents work through different mechanisms, but the ultimate brain systems responsible for modulating anxious states still are under study. However, a great deal is not yet known about the chemistry of anxiety and the mechanisms responsible for it. Much focus has been centered on the limbic system, one of the most primitive parts of the brain that modulates emotions. A neurotransmitter called gamma-aminobutyric acid (GABA) almost certainly has an important role in the actions of the benzodi-azepines and buspirone. There are specific sites on receptors in the brain where GABA acts and to which the benzodizap-ines attach. How that causes such a profound change in anxiety levels, however, remains to be seen.

Side Effects

Antihistamines are relatively well tolerated over a wide range of doses. Sedation and daytime drowsiness are common side effects, as well as dry mouth and possibly blurry vision. As for the benzodiazepines, they are remarkably safe. If injected intravenously too rapidly, they can cause breathing to stop, but doses many times higher than those typically used for medical purposes are unlikely to do more than cause the patient to sleep for several hours. The most common side effects with appropriate use are sedation, daytime drowsiness, and a decrease in mental sharpness. There also is the risk of behavioral disinhibition in children.

Doctors and parents should be alert to possible abuse by children or adolescents who are taking a benzodiazapene. This involves monitoring the child's supply of the medication and being certain all pills are appropriately accounted for. However, abuse typically occurs after months or years, not days or weeks.

The beta-adrenergic antagonists, such as propranolol, require more caution, although they, too, are typically well tolerated. With increasing doses, they can slow the heart rate and lower blood pressure; these effects account for their efficacy in treating high blood pressure and certain types of heart diseases. They can also cause sedation and drowsiness, especially at fairly high doses.

Buspirone is remarkable for a relative absence of serious side effects.

Using Antianxiety Medications

The key to the successful use of these medications is not to wait until the last minute. If you have a child with a developmental delay who hates being stuck in an airplane for hours but has to fly, then it may be useful to consider diphenhydramine or even a benzodiazepine. What you don't want to do is wait until you are already on the airplane to try the medicine for the very first time. You probably won't know the right dose, and children who are already upset seem much more likely to resist the calming effects of these drugs and are probably more likely to become disinhibited.

To start, try a dose or two well before the trip to get an idea what dosage you need and how long it will last. Give your child the medication on a day when you

REASONS FOR USING ANTIDEPRESSANTS
IN CHILDREN AND ADOLESCENTS

DISORDERS

> Anxiety disorders, especially with panic attacks

SEVERE BEHAVIORS

> Acute grief or bereavement reactions

> Acute trauma

> Transient problems getting to sleep (onset insomnia)

> Major disruptions associated with a specific event such as air travel or a medical or dental procedure

. . . .

are with him or her, so you can monitor the effects and how long they last. This will provide you with the information you need to judge when and how often your child may need to be medicated.

In general, oral medications such as pills take anywhere from twenty to forty minutes to begin working; liquids may work faster. Pills dissolved under the tongue (make sure the medicine isn't so bitter that the child will spit it out) can work even faster, but they still take time.

Similarly, if a child is having serious trouble getting to sleep after a traumatic event, a brief course of an antihistamine such as diphenhydramine may be worth considering. If so, make sure you add in other rituals to encourage sleep and give

the medicine a half an hour or so before bedtime. Letting the child run around the house at top speed until he is exhausted is not a good strategy. After giving him the pill, encourage him to engage in a quiet activity until it is time to turn out the light—a warm bath followed by soothing music are good strategies. Ultimately, such activities should supersede the need for a medication.

Guidelines for Using Diphenhydramine

Diphenhydramine (Benadryl) is available without a prescription, and parents often already have some experience with its effectiveness in treating allergy and cold symptoms. It is calming and sedating and

MORE THAN ONE WAY TO HELP

At age twelve, Allan began having increasingly debilitating problems with anxiety, phobias, and panic attacks. It started with a few simple fears, mainly that someone might break into the house while the family slept, which began when he heard about a burglary in the neighborhood. Gradually, his fears expanded. At least twice each evening he needed to make sure every window and door in the house was locked before he could go to bed, and he sometimes awoke during the night and would check them all again. Unlike someone with OCD, Allan justified his checking as reasonable and reassuring, even though he admitted it might be a little excessive.

Otherwise, Allan had excellent grades, close friends who thought he was a bit "kooky" but rarely teased him, and an intact family. He began to suspect he needed help when he started dreading being out of the house because someone might break in while the house was empty. Then he had his first panic attack: As he walked out the door to go to school one morning, Allan was suddenly overcome with a sense of impending doom, his heart was pounding so hard that he was sure it would burst, and he abruptly became dizzy. He was convinced that he was about to die. His parents rushed him to the emergency room, where the staff found nothing physically wrong but noticed that he was hyperventilating (breathing too rapidly), which was making him dizzy. They had him breathe in a paper bag and gave him a dose of lorazepam (Ativan).

By the time I saw Allan several weeks later, he'd had five more panic attacks, each ending in a visit to the emergency room. He readily described what had been happening and said he knew nothing was wrong with his heart, yet asked soon thereafter, "But what if there is?" After educating Allan about anxiety and panic attacks, we agreed on a plan. We decided that he should keep lorazepam with him all the time in case he felt a panic attack coming on. This helped reduce the lengths of his panic attacks, and his visits to the emergency room stopped. At the same time, Allan also started taking a low-dose SSRI, after I explained that it would have little immediate benefit but that after several weeks it should lower his anxiety level and make his panic attacks less frequent and intense.

Finally, we started an extinction program to help Allan overcome his constant checking behaviors. As his anxiety reduced, he found that increasingly easy to do. Within three months, he was free of panic attacks, but kept the lorazepam with him at all times for another three months, just in case. By then, he had also significantly reduced his checking behaviors. His friends still liked him—and still thought he was kooky.

has long been a favorite initial treatment, even in child psychiatric inpatient units, for dealing with severe tantrums and rages. It is safe and well-tolerated over a fairly wide dose range, with the most common limiting side effect of putting the patient to sleep. However, it also causes dry mouth, daytime sleepiness, and confusion.

Diphenhydramine can be handy for parents with easily overwhelmed children with time-limited problems such as severe sleep disturbances after moving to a new house or the inability to tolerate a long flight. Some children with developmental delays such as mental retardation or autism are stable as long as they have their routines but can become transiently overwhelmed by seemingly minor stress; diphenhydramine can also be helpful for them.

Diphenhydramine is available in a range of preparations, including liquid, pills, and capsules. Doses range from 12.5 mg to 50 mg, depending on the child's age and response, and can be repeated several times a day if needed. Again, it is best to give the medication before problems begin, and the need to use it repeatedly over more than a few days probably means you should see a professional.

Sleeping Pills

All of us have, at some point in our lives, had a night or two where it has been tough getting to sleep or staying asleep. Personally, every time I travel I can count on at least one night of far too little sleep—and it doesn't even seem to matter whether I'm going west to east or east to west. Similarly, stress at school, work, or just too much excitement in one's life may manifest as sleeplessness.

Taking substances to promote sleep has to be one of the oldest uses of medicines, if you consider warm milk and hot toddies. Many medications have sedative properties, so marketing products for that purpose also have a long and illustrious history. Unfortunately, a number of medications work fine if you have a temporary problem with getting to sleep—but so does doing nothing. If you look at over-the-counter sleeping aids, most are antihistamines or anticholinergics. They work for a few nights but become less effective over time, and increased doses lead to more side effects, including daytime drowsiness, decreased motor coordination, and slowed thinking and reflexes.

Chronic sleep disturbances are the more difficult problems that adults and parents bring to physicians. Sleep disturbances are often a symptom of another problem, so the preferred method of treating that insomnia is to work on the root problem. For example, if sedation is the goal, one can either use a sedating antidepressant to give prompt relief or a nonsedating antidepressant with the expectation that sleep will improve as the depression lifts.

But what about regular sleep disorders? They do indeed occur, but with a few exceptions there are essentially no studies of the use of medication to treat such problems in children. Sleep disturbances break down into problems getting to sleep (onset insomnia), staying asleep (middle insomnia or sleep disruptions such as nightmares or sleep walking), and waking up too early (late insomnia).

The great bulk of research (almost exclusively in adults) is on onset insomnia, and most marketed medications, prescription or over-the-counter, focus on getting people to sleep. In my experience, that is why parents rarely seek a doctor's help with their child. Adolescents often have horrible sleep patterns; they stay up too late and have trouble getting up when they need to. Medications are seldom appropriate, or even wanted, in these situations. With younger children, sleep-onset problems typically have to do with anxiety issues and can be handled behaviorally. Behavioral interventions are less helpful for middle-onset disturbances or early-morning wakening.

The true age of the sleeping pill began in the 1970s, with the search for a safe medication that produces natural, restful sleep with no daytime side effects. This

has proven difficult to attain. The first widely used medication marked specifically as a sleeping pill was flurazepam (Dalmane), a benzodiazepine. Some years later, it was supplanted with triazolam (Halcion), also a benzodiazepine. Both were successful at getting people to sleep, but they tended to have cumulative effects when used chronically, with the potential for slowing thinking processes and reflexes during the day without the user being aware of the change.

A new group of non-benzodiazpine sleeping pills have become available over the past few years (see table on antianxiety agents used in children and adolescents). In adults, they seem less likely to produce daytime side effects, but chronic use still is discouraged. There is no systematic experience with them in children and adolescents.

For the past several years, melatonin, a brain neurotransmitter in the pineal gland, has become a popular natural sleeping agent. Research (including in children), seems to suggest that it can be especially helpful for sleep problems that arise because of time shifts such as traveling across time zones or during daylight saving time. There are suggestions that the effect wears off with time, making chronic use not appropriate. Of more concern is the fact that melatonin is treated as a supplement and therefore not under FDA scrutiny. A few years ago reports stated that some over-the-counter preparations of melatonin actually contained an anticholinergic drug.

In my practice, I usually consider using medications for two types of sleep problems. The first are children with mental retardation or autism who wake up in the middle of the night, ready for a new day. They are a danger to themselves and others, because they may waken without alerting other family members. I've heard stories of parents finding their child awake and into things in the middle of the night. Even worse are parents who receive a call late at night from a concerned neighbor who's noticed that their autistic child is wandering down the street, completely naked and obviously lost. I typically use trazodone (Desyrel) for these children, because its major side effect is sedation, and sleep studies have suggested the type of sleep trazodone induces is relatively similar to natural sleep. Doses range from 25 to 300 mg or more, depending on the age and size of the child.

Second, and fortunately much rarer, are those children who have severe and sustained night terrors. Kris, whom I treated many years ago, is still among the youngest children I have prescribed a medication for. He was three-and-a-half years old when the behavioral team working with him and his family finally gave up. He'd been having major sleep problems for nine months, and resisted going to sleep because he feared the terrifying dreams he would have, often several times a night. Each time, Kris would cry inconsolably for thirty minutes or more before finally waking up, and then do his best to stay awake to avoid a repeat. He and his parents were getting by on three hours or less of sleep a night.

Night terrors still are not completely understood, but it is known that the disruption of certain phases of sleep could be helpful and imipramine, a tricyclic antidepressant, produced that kind of disruption. Almost as if by magic, Kris slept through the night the second night we gave him a low dose of imipramine. He continued to do well as long as he took the imipramine but, when we tried to wean him off the medicine at age five, his night terrors promptly returned. I sent him to a sleep disorders clinic, which failed to find a reason for his difficulty, but took over his care.

The Bottom Line

In my experience, antianxiety agents have limited use in children. Although many are relatively safe, regular use can cause problems, so chronic reliance on them is not advised. Other medication strategies, especially antidepressants, are typically more satisfactory in the long run.

Still, these medications can be of great value in certain emergency situations, and short-term usage seems to carry little risk. They often are also highly useful companions to other medications, lessening side effects and adding benefits, at relatively low doses and for limited periods.

These principles hold equally for the use of medications that treat sleep problems. I generally work hard with parents to find other ways of helping their children get the rest they need without medications. If they have a problem that is likely to pass after a few days, I may suggest a short course of diphenhydramine or melatonin, both available without a prescription. Beyond that, the need for medication must be clear, with no evidence of a treatable underlying disorder.

PART FOUR

Looking Beyond Medications

Each of these chapters has a different focus, but all are intended to provide a view beyond the medical model of disorders and medications.

Chapter 13 describes a range of treatments aside from medications that are commonly used for various childhood psychiatric disorders. Discussing them together in a single chapter is in no way intended to suggest either that they are all alike or less useful than medications. In fact, several of the treatments described here are favored interventions for some illnesses. However, this is a book about medications, so I leave more extensive descriptions of the specific methods to others.

Chapter 13 also includes a sampling of the array of commonly used alternative treatments. Even though I am skeptical about many of them, I have had enough parents tell me tales of success about controversial treatments to know the power of the promise they make for cures, or at least gains. Beyond sharing with you what available evidence tells us about some of these treatments, I strive mainly to suggest guidelines to help you to decide if your child is actually benefiting from these treatments.

Chapter 14 addresses some of the common issues you might face with schools if your child had a psychiatric disorder. School can either be a source of incredible frustration, an invaluable resource, or both. You have the power to play a role in enhancing the usefulness of teachers and other school personnel while diminishing the frustrations that arise due to the tension between meeting the needs of one child while fulfilling the broader mandate of educating all children.

Finally, Chapter 15 explores why I wrote this book. It contains nothing new, nor do I try to recapitulate key concepts. Save it for last. Most of all, it is my effort to honor you, the parents of incredibly precious children with unbelievably difficult problems that you all must face together.

Chapter 13

Nondrug Therapies

For the large majority of children who need treatment, medications are only a part of the answer. Complex conditions typically require complex treatments, and many children can benefit from therapies beyond the medications described here. Such interventions break down into several broad categories: psychotherapies, "natural" treatments such as vitamins and other supplements, and somatic treatments that on focus "correcting" parts of the body that are "out of order." Some of these treatments are well-studied and have clear proof of benefit, while others have a long history of use with variable levels of evidence for safety and efficacy. Still others seem to materialize overnight, gain considerable popularity with minimal or no objective support, and then disappear almost as rapidly as they appeared.

Like the medicine men who traveled America, selling potions to their audiences for whatever ailed them, there are always people looking for a way to make money. In many cases, anecdotal success by doctors or laypeople became the basis for the marshaling of great numbers of believers. Some of these methods lack any sort of validity, yet they still drain families of financial and emotional resources.

As explained in previous chapters, medical practitioners need to be creative in their use of prescription medications for children, since so few have actually been tested on this age group. How then, does that differ from these other approaches? The answer is: Not nearly enough, and a great deal. We, too, can fool ourselves. Look at the recent rush to embrace the new generation of antipsychotics—their unique risks are only now becoming clear. Learning from these changes and expanding our knowledge base makes a big difference. If you find a treatment that you are told is perfectly safe, universally effective for a wide range of disorders, and "ignored" or "actively suppressed" by the medical establishment, then you have probably discovered something that is, in fact, too good to be true. However, speaking both for myself and for my professional colleagues, I am not so beholden to the pharmaceutical companies that I would pass up a genuine nondrug cure for ADHD, autism, or any other severe disorder.

Psychotherapy

Psychotherapy is an extremely broad term that describes a relationship in which a patient seeks help for a mental illness or emotional problems from a person who has expertise in offering such help. Such a person might be a psychiatrist, psychologist, social worker, religious counselor, or even a lay therapist (someone with no formal training). The patient may be seeking more information about a disorder or problem (educational psychotherapy), sympathy and assistance for self or family (supportive psychotherapy), or insights or tools for dealing with a disorder or behavioral problem (interventional psychotherapy). The focus of the therapy also can vary according to individual, parent, or group. The format for sessions may range from simple talking to various forms of play to experiential therapy, such as role-play or drama. Duration can vary from a few sessions to intense workshops to frequent meetings over many years.

Types of Therapy

Behavior Modification

Behavior modification is rooted in cogni-tive behavior therapy. It posits that a child's behavior is responsive to influences from the environment, and that deliberate changes in that environment (at home or school, for example) can alter a child's functioning. A specially trained teacher or a mental health professional will most likely set up a behavior modification program. In some situations, the goal is to eliminate a negative behavior; at other times, the point is to teach the child a new, positive behavior. Goals can be as simple as teaching a child to come to the table at dinnertime, or it can be a complex series of steps that will help an ADHD child better approach homework or a autistic child learn how to interact with others.

The keys to behavior modification are to set achievable goals that the child can accomplish and to get responsible adults, including parents, teachers, grandparents, and other caregivers to apply the required behavioral interventions regularly and consistently. Once the plan and goals are set, it is essential for the new behavior to be expected and rewarded by all who interact with the child.

If you are setting up a behavior modification program for your child, here are some key points to keep in mind:

• **Agree on target behaviors.** Targeted behaviors must be very specific: "obeys teacher request when first asked" or "does not hit sibling." "Learn to be good" is too vague—specificity is key.

- **Try to replace negative behaviors with incompatible neutral or positive ones.** For example, if the negative behavior is thumb-sucking, consider having the child keep that hand in her pocket when not otherwise occupied.
- **Agree upon the type of reward with the child.** Parents often object to bribing their child, yet feel just fine about accepting a bonus at work for high productivity. Rewards don't have to be extravagant, but they must be meaningful and timely. Younger children need immediate rewards; older children may have some capacity for long-term rewards but may benefit from a marker, such as a chart, to monitor progress.
- **Use appropriate commands.** Work out simple, consistent instructions. Don't confuse the child with too much detail or multiple instructions.
- **Discuss what happens if the child doesn't cooperate.** Negative consequences may be needed if the child doesn't cooperate, but should be phased out as quickly as possible and must be reasonable enough that you do not feel guilty applying them, and thereby sabotage the effort.
- **Start small, then build on success.** If the target is not hitting a sibling, focus first on specific times of day or situations where the behavior is most often a problem, then expand into other settings that may be harder to monitor or intervene.
- **Keep it simple and manageable.** Charts and chore-reward systems can be wonderful, but only if you have the time and energy to enforce them.

The hardest part of behavioral programs, oddly enough, is often keeping them going after the initial success. Often, families are delighted with their child's response to a behavioral program but then drop it soon after the problem behavior has diminished and then are disappointed when the behavior suddenly reemerges. Imagine breaking a leg and getting a cast— would you take it off the next day just because you were back on your feet? Behavioral programs take time to cause permanent changes, and sometimes they must be maintained indefinitely.

Cognitive Behavior Therapies

Cognitive behavior therapies are among the more vigorously researched of all areas of psychotherapy, with good evidence of benefit for a number of major childhood and adolescent mental disorders. This type of therapy treats a number of mental disorders through the systematic application of well-established principles that connect thoughts with actions, and has proven effective for several anxiety disorders, particularly panic disorder and social phobia; OCD; depression; and ADHD. A variant also appears to be effective in treating the core symptoms of autism in a select group of patients. Generally, for younger children (typically below about age eight), practitioners work mainly with parents and other caregivers to help them better understand how the child's behaviors manifest and teach them behavioral modification techniques. With older children and adolescents, the child often becomes a more active participant in the process, learning not only about their illness but also techniques for changing behaviors themselves.

For example, a cognitive behavioral therapist helping a child overcome a fear of starting a new school might guide the child toward focusing on developing the necessary tools for greeting a new situation optimistically. Depending on the age of the child, these tools might involve anything from reminding a younger child that the question, "Can I play?" will often be answered affirmatively to discussing strategies with a thirteen-year-old girl who may find herself eating alone on the first few days of school. A therapist might also help a child with a phobia of dogs overcome this fear by first showing the child photographs of dogs, then watching and discussing a movie with a dog in it, and then eventually exposing the child, under controlled circumstances, to reliable, trustworthy pets. As the child becomes more comfortable with these situations, the therapist might eventually expose the child to random dogs on the street. For a child with OCD who is spending prolonged periods of time tidying, a therapist might help her leave one corner of her room disordered for a day. The therapist would then also help the child work through the resulting feelings of anxiety.

To be effective, this therapy requires active cooperation by the family and the child. It is hard work, and typically includes specific tasks and considerable practice. To effectively mold behaviors in a positive direction, it must be applied with consistency and sufficient understanding of the child and disorder. Like any potent intervention, misuse can lead to deterioration of behavior rather than improvement. This type of therapy also offers tools that may be applicable to other conditions that may arise.

A relatively new variation of cognitive behavior therapy, called dialectical behavior therapy (DBT), has gained positive attention for its success in dealing with adolescents who have suicidal thoughts or who harm themselves (usually by burning or cutting). The overall structure remains focused on thinking, but focuses more attention on the effects of emotional states on behavior than traditional cognitive techniques. DBT encourages the individual to take responsibility for their behavior and develop ways to cope with the negative feelings that create it.

Medication is often combined with cognitive behavior therapy to help a child get started on the program. However, some experts urge patients or families to try the behavioral approach first, since it is less useful if the medication effectively wipes out the problematic behaviors. Originally, cognitive behavioral therapies were intended to be relatively brief, typically multiple sessions over several months. However, some forms of therapy in this class may require ongoing interventions of indefinite duration, leaving families responsible for judging whether they continue to be of value.

Dynamic Therapies

Dynamic therapies focus on the theory that current behaviors arise from past events and that the best, and possibly only, way to change current behavior is through an understanding of that connection. There are a number of schools of dynamic thought, but all based on the research of Sigmund Freud at the turn of the twentieth century. He focused largely on adults, but others, including his daughter, Anna Freud, extended the method into adolescence and childhood.

Much of the original basis of dynamic therapy came from intensive work with relatively few patients who were seen up to six times a week for many years. These interactions produced rich observations about how the mind works, but less intense interventions have yet to show the same benefit. Now, much dynamic work is done with weekly (or even less frequent) therapy and sometimes with a limited number of total sessions. Seeing the success of time-limited cognitive therapies, researchers have developed a manual that teaches a clinician to offer insight-oriented treatment for depression. This intervention, called interpersonal therapy (IPT), has proven effective in adults and holds promise for some types of adolescent depression.

However, distorting any intervention too much can mean losing the elements that made it successful in the first place. As with anything else, when research is lacking, the risk grows greater. Dynamic principles have influenced child mental health since the inception of the field in the mid-1950s. A challenge for the field, and for you as a parent, is to determine whether dynamic therapy as applied in most settings today remains helpful and, if so, for what disorders and which patients.

Therapy Settings

Individual Therapies

As the name implies, individual therapies entail work between a single patient and a trained therapist. This is not so much a type of therapy as a style. Depending on the therapist's training, work may range from educational to supportive to interventional to a mix of all of them (often called "eclectic"). A dynamic therapist might help the child or adolescent try to understand current problems on the basis of past events, such as problems with parenting, major losses, or other developmental issues. A cognitive therapist might look more at current behaviors and help the patient shape them along more desirable lines. The underlying theme here is that the individual is responsible for his or her

---

PLAY THERAPY

For many years, play therapy was the sole type of intervention for younger children, almost regardless of diagnosis. It was the subject of little research, both because those who used it believed in its efficacy and because it is hard to standardize such an approach in a way that makes research easy. Play therapy has been criticized—justly in my opinion—as easily becoming simply a part of the child's weekly routine, with little to no evidence of benefit. Parents may also feel especially conflicted because the child comes home after each session saying, "We just played." Indeed, for certain disorders including anxiety disorders, OCD, and ADHD, available research suggests that play therapy has little to no benefit.

Even though play therapy's role in treating mental illness is under question, it still remains a key part of our child and adolescent psychiatry training program at UCSF. It can offer a rich window into the life of a child. For example, a nearly three-year-old sweet, intelligent girl with whom I had brief contact many years ago had been hospitalized many times for physical problems deliberately caused by her mother (a disorder called Munchausen's syndrome by proxy). Direct questioning produced little information from this shy but cooperative child. However, during play therapy, she was immediately drawn to a toy doctor's kit, and began repeatedly injecting her mother with a toy syringe, saying, "This won't hurt a bit." It turned out the mother had been giving her daughter insulin shots, which caused her blood sugar to plummet. The little girl also found a small, colored cube that she tried to get the therapist to pretend to eat, saying, "Umm-umm, this is good candy!" Her mother had also been giving her a laxative that looked like the cube.

---

behavior and can make changes that will have positive results.

With younger children, especially those before puberty, individual therapy that focuses on talking can be highly unproductive. Few four- or five-year-olds have the cognitive and language skills needed to engage in a thoughtful discussion about their behaviors and how to change them. Many years ago, therapists showed that play can be a highly productive avenue for accessing the child's thoughts and feelings and even perhaps for helping that child learn new ways of thinking and dealing with painful or difficult feelings. Again, there are many different ways in which such play therapy can be utilized, depending on the therapist's school of training.

Certain kinds of behavioral or experiential problems also may be helped by play therapy, although the evidence is not conclusive. Some researchers have shown that children recently traumatized by an accident or natural disaster may be able to work through their fears and function better by playing out the problems and gradually introducing alternative outcomes and solutions.

One of the long-standing criticisms of play therapy, and many other forms of individual therapy, is that they are not time-limited. When parents or the child ask how long the therapy will last, they may receive no real answer. Too often, the answer is when there is no money left or the family or therapist decides to move on to a different therapy.

My advice to families and adolescents engaged in individual therapy is to ask the therapist to discuss what the therapy is designed to help, how everyone can judge its success, and when it is reasonable to measure benefit.

Family Therapies

Family therapies also embody a wide range of underlying schools of thought, with a central hypothesis that certain mental disorders or behavioral problems may manifest in a single individual but are a direct result of, or at least are heavily influenced by, disturbances in the entire household. The appropriate intervention then, should be with the family, not the identified patient, who is merely providing evidence of the disturbance. For instance, a child with a severe eating disorder may be providing a way for the parents, who have intense but unexpressed conflicts with each other, to stay together, for the sake of the child. Family therapy attempts to identify the underlying disturbances and help the family function in a more positive manner by improving communication and providing education and support about the issues the family is facing.

After the therapist has evaluated the situation, he or she recommends how the sessions should be constructed. The therapist may want to include the child along with the parents, siblings, and grandparents (if they are part of the household), or see certain members of the family separately. Family therapy can be particularly helpful in cases of divorce or when a couple cannot agree on how to deal with the child or who constantly blame one child while ignoring problems other siblings are having.

Effective family therapy requires a well-trained and competent therapist. It is hard to work with a number of people and the complexity of the interactions that arise. Family therapy is often used as an adjunct to other types of therapy, frequently with a different therapist than the one working with the child individually.

Group Therapies

This form of therapy uses group dynamics and peer interactions to deal with problem behaviors. The underlying school of thought may be dynamic, cognitive, educational, or supportive, but the uniting assumption is that the patient, parents, or whole family will learn best by sharing knowledge with others, usually peers. Thus, a child with ADHD might engage in group therapy to explore ways of socially interacting better with peers. In a cognitive-based approach, the child might first learn about the steps of greeting a new peer and then practice the newly taught skill with an actual peer, probably another child with ADHD. A videotape of that interaction might help the whole group see what worked and what didn't.

Some cognitively based interventions, such as DBT for self-injurious teenagers, seem to work well in a group setting. Basic information is efficiently conveyed in programmed modules for up to eight to ten patients at a time, and the adolescents can reinforce their newly learned skills by testing them out on each other.

Group therapy has a mixed status in the U.S. Patients and families often fear that it is a poor substitute to individual therapy. In some cases, that judgment may be correct. However, as with the example of ADHD and social skills, evidence is showing that sometimes peer pressure and real-time application of skills that group settings facilitate may be superior for certain kinds of interventions.

"Natural" Treatments and Supplements

Special Diets

Special diets have long been an area of intense interest to parents with children who have serious mental disorders, especially ADHD and autism. In the early 1970s, a Kaiser pediatric allergist in San Francisco became convinced that a number of behavioral problems, including ADHD, were the result of allergic reactions to certain artificial additives found in processed foods (salicylates, certain artificial colors and flavors, and artificial sweeteners, to name a few). Restricting such substances reportedly led to significant behavioral benefits. Such dietary approaches remain quite popular, despite the enormous effort involved in successfully avoiding all the proscribed substances. Research in the area still remains controversial, although my interpretation of the available studies suggests that the problem, to the extent that there is one, is worse in younger children and grows less after age six or seven.

Diets that restrict exposure to gluten and casein, substances found in the seeds of various cereal grains, are also popular. There is a well-defined disorder, called celiac sprue, in which individuals develop gastrointestinal symptoms and other problems as a result of poor tolerance of these substances. The controversy lies in whether such a problem causes or worsens the symptoms of autism. Complete avoidance of all such grains is enormously difficult for families, and I have met few for whom the result was a clear reversal of the symptoms of autism.

Nutritional Supplements

Nutritional supplements come in a range of forms that have in common the belief that certain childhood mental disorders, including ADHD, autism, and bipolar disorder, are helped with the addition of large amounts of vitamins or other naturally occurring substances. A recent example of this is the use of fish oils as a mood stabilizer. Many products combine a range of rare minerals and essential vitamins in high doses, with claims of great success for various disorders. All of these preparations are outside the jurisdiction of the FDA, because the U.S. Congress explicitly excluded them from the scrutiny that prescription medications must undergo for safety and efficacy. I am highly skeptical of the claims products of this type make but have no hard evidence of either efficacy or inefficacy.

Somatic Treatments

Electroconvulsive Therapy

Electroconvulsive therapy (ECT) is a highly controversial, but quite old, intervention that is mainly used for treating severe, treatment-resistant depression and psychotic illnesses. It is rarely used in children but is sometimes recommended for adolescents who have failed to respond to medication. First utilized for severe mental disorders in the 1930s, the acceptability of ECT has varied widely over the years. Improvements in the way it is administered have made it safer and less likely to produce lasting adverse side effects, but there is still no real understanding of how it works. Still, evidence has shown that it can be helpful in severe illnesses for which nothing else has helped.

Transcranial Magnetic Stimulation

This treatment method is a noninvasive, outpatient procedure for depression that

---

ADDITIONAL QUESTIONS

If you are going to a psychotherapist or are seriously considering investing in an alternative treatment as part of your plan to help your child, many of the suggestions made earlier concerning connecting with the right professional still apply. If you are making a long-term commitment to therapy for your child, clear up any insurance issues right away. Few people want, or are able, to pay regular therapy bills entirely out-of-pocket.

In addition, personal chemistry may be very crucial. Some studies, of both individual and group therapy, suggest that the single most important factor in determining outcome is the relationship between the therapist and patient. Carefully evaluate your own, and your child's, comfort level with the person. Do you like the way they interact with your child? Does your child seem comfortable with him or her? And how do you feel when the professional gives you feedback? If the whole family is involved, it may be difficult to find someone who pleases everyone, but you should certainly be aware if one or two family members are particularly resistant to the therapist.

It may be helpful to ask the following questions:

- What training and experience have you had in treating this type of disorder?
- What is your basic approach?
- How frequent are sessions, and how long do they last?
- How long is the course of treatment?
- How will we know when the treatment is done?
- Do you include other family members in the process?
- Do you accept health insurance?

has resisted other treatments. It has just received approval from the FDA and is already being used in Canada, Australia, and Israel. The process works by delivering pulses of magnetic energy to the left or right of the prefrontal cortex of the brain, which is involved with regulating mood. The patient is not sedated for the procedure, which takes about thirty to forty-five minutes and uses a magnetic coil on the scalp to send a painless, five-second pulse to the appropriate part of the brain in thirty-second intervals. Its usefulness in children and adolescents still requires further study.

Questionable Therapies

EEG Training

EEG training is a therapy recommended especially for ADHD, and posits that children can learn to alter certain types of EEG activity through biofeedback, an assertion that may be true. By learning how to increase "calm" EEG patterns, the patient can learn to control inattention, impulsivity, and hyperactivity. Some studies suggest that children who successfully alter their EEG patterns in the prescribed fashion show improvements in the laboratory setting. What no studies have been able to demonstrate is if such laboratory changes

make a difference at home or in school. Such effects would be crucial for this treatment to be truly effective.

Holding Therapy

Holding therapy is an intervention that became popular in the 1990s as a way to increase attachment with a child. It was originally created as a way to work with autistic adults, and it was then applied to autistic children as well as to adolescents and younger children with attachment disorders. Later on it was applied to infants with residual birth trauma. Parents of adopted children and families where the parents felt the child was detached began implementing it as well, based on advice in *Holding Time*, a book by Martha G. Welch. The theory that holding a child until he stops resisting or initiates eye contact can treat autism or any other form of attachment problem is highly controversial. The therapy has its advocates, but the procedure is exhausting and requires careful controls to ensure the safety of the child and parent, especially with adolescents and larger children. No controlled studies have demonstrated efficacy.

Chelation Therapy

Chelation therapy involves a prescription medication that induces the removal of minerals from the body. The use of this alternative therapy for autism has captured public interest, although anecdotal reports have failed to withstand the rigors of actual research. These reports suggest that autism might be a result of toxicity caused by mercury, introduced into children either as a preservative in vaccines or through contamination in foods such as farm-raised salmon.

Scientists now have convincingly refuted a link between the mercury in vaccinations and the rise in autism, so parents who seek out chelation as a form of therapy are probably following a false lead for a false reason. The chelation process encourages the body to shed its metal content, but the drugs can also cause liver and kidney damage and remove beneficial minerals such as zinc, copper, and iron, making supplements necessary. Bimonthly blood tests are also required in order to follow the progress of the therapy.

Chelation therapy is approved by the FDA, but only when blood tests reveal heavy-metal poisoning.

Homeopathy

Homeopathy is one of the most intriguing and baffling of the alternative therapies. It asserts that certain substances and disorders are connected to each other, so tiny amounts of the former (dilutions of one part per million or even one part per billion) can cause improvements in the latter. Thus, if hyperactivity is the target, essence of bumblebee might be useful in treating it. Homeopaths prepare an individually tailored solution consisting of water, a few molecules of bumblebee extract, and several other animals or plant extracts that also have affinities for the specific behaviors the child exhibits. Research on this treatment for childhood mental disorders is quite sparse.

Emerging Alternative Remedies

New theories on children and mental illness emerge regularly, especially in the realm of alternative therapies. While this book explores traditional forms of treatment, I am well aware that new theories and treatments are becoming available all the time, and so may not be included here.

For the most part, tried and true options are that way for a reason. Most of topics discussed here have some level of FDA approval; even those medications not specifically approved for children have been approved for human use, and they have held up under years of scrutiny by prescribing physicians. For these treatments, there is knowledge of what works and what doesn't.

That said, a promising intervention

will inevitably present itself. I would never tell anyone to ignore their intuition and refuse to consider any intervention they think might benefit their child. What I do recommend is that the possible benefits be weighed against the possible risk.

If you are trying an alternative intervention, be sure to learn answers to the following questions:

- **How are treatments evaluated?** Are there any scientific studies of the process? A rigorous medical study will likely be published in a scientific journal, and this would be a significant piece of evidence for an acceptable treatment. If all proof of success is anecdotal, be cautious. Patient or doctor testimonials do not mean that the process is harmful; it just means there is no real proof.

- **Have clinical trials been conducted demonstrating the efficacy and safety of the process?** The absence of this evidence may reflect many factors, but the existence of clinical research gives you much more information about the treatment.

- **Are any results published in peer-reviewed journals?** Beware of in-house publications, sometimes quite lavishly prepared, which are truly only fancy advertisements.

- **Is information on the process available from the National Center for Complementary and Alternative Medicine (NCCAM) at the National Institute of Health?** This center supports research on alternative medicine, and their support is not necessarily official approval, but it is a good sign. The office can be reached toll-free at 888-644-6226 or through its Web site at http://nccam.nih.gov.

- **Is there a national organization or state licensing of practitioners?** As interventions and practitioners mature, oversight organizations tend to arise to assure quality and help highlight less reputable businesses.

- **Is treatment reimbursed by health insurance?** Insurance coverage certainly does not establish the efficacy or inefficacy of a treatment, but it may affect its affordability.

Unfortunately, you need to develop a healthy skepticism for what you read in the press, especially reports on new treatments—and not just for mental illnesses. Look closely at news reports about a brand-new intervention, and you will often find only one or two sources for the story and no mention of the involvement of a medical school, a national organization, or a government agency. This doesn't mean the treatment is bad, just unproven, and it remains to be seen whether it is good or bad.

Chapter 14

Working with Your Child's School

School is an incredibly important part of growing up, as we may recall from our own childhood. It constitutes the major environment outside of the home and family for exposure to peers and adults who are part of the wider world. For better or worse, most of us remember at least one particularly influential teacher—hopefully because they were nurturing us and not bent on bringing us down.

Children with serious mental disorders often have particular needs that must be in place so they can perform to the best of their ability at school. Furthermore, schools are obligated by law to provide all children with educational opportunities and services. This chapter discusses the issues that commonly arise with schools when a child has a major mental illness, whether or not medication is part of the treatment. Parents can help create the right school environment for their child by understanding their family's legal rights and establishing clear lines of communications between home and school. These elements are crucial for optimal treatment of any child with an emotional or behavioral disorder.

Unfortunately, not all parents have adopted this philosophy, to the detriment of their child. Some fear their child will be rejected if they reveal that he has psychological problems, so they resist telling school officials about medication or that he is seeing a doctor. Such a decision can deprive the child of much-needed services and disconnect the family from potentially valuable perspectives of the child's behavior.

Gwen, a twelve-year-old with moderate ADHD, serves as an example of what happens when parents do not communicate with their child's school. Her parents kept her off her stimulant all summer because they were worried about her appetite. Although this period was sometimes rough, the family decided Gwen had done well enough, and they wanted to see if she still needed the stimulant at all. Since Gwen was starting the sixth grade in a new middle school, they decided to not tell her new teachers about her ADHD and see if they noticed. All went smoothly at first, although her parents were surprised at how little homework Gwen seemed to have. The plan failed completely at midterm, when four of her five teachers sent home notices (only two made it home) indicating that their previously excellent student was getting Ds and Fs. Even after she went back on her stimulant, several of Gwen's teachers were convinced that she didn't really apply herself as a student, and her grades suffered.

Other parents have refused to grant me permission to even contact their child's school. Some have insisted that I avoid revealing the child's actual diagnosis. I have had children with autism whose parents wanted me to give a diagnosis of anxiety so the children would not be stigmatized. Clear communication between the educational and mental health systems can be difficult enough without deliberate obfuscation of what is wrong with a child and what is being done about it.

If your child is not yet in school, he or she is still entitled to early intervention educational support. There is more information regarding children under age five later in this chapter.

The Law Is on Your Side

Whether your child has a physical, psychiatric, emotional, or behavior disorder, or a learning disability, federal law in the U.S. mandates that every child receive a free and appropriate education in an appropriate environment. It also entitles children with special needs to receive extra services, although there is no requirement for schools to provide optimal school environments, only adequate ones.

Whether a child is in a separate setting or is mainstreamed in the regular classroom and receives extra services there will vary from state to state and child to child. Some states have specified that as many children as possible should be in the regular classroom; others favor having separate classes for the more seriously disabled and mainstreaming them only for physical education and the arts. Such preferences vary with time and administrative beliefs, so you will need to explore the specifics of your child's situation. Also, the provision of special accommodations is the responsibility of public schools; private schools tend either to specialize in children with learning or behavioral problems, typically at an increased cost, or to refuse to accept them altogether.

Special accommodations to aid in learning may include some of the following services: untimed testing, front-of-the-class seat assignments, modified homework, structured learning environment, verbal instructions on test-taking in addition to written ones, use of tape recorders or computer-aided learning processes, behavioral management techniques, access to nursing services for medication, counseling or other forms of therapy, or other necessary services. Though criteria for eligibility and level of services vary from state to state, parents should have a general understanding of all the laws and regulations.

Individual with Disabilities Education Act

The Individuals with Disabilities Education Act (IDEA) is a federal law governing all special education services for children. It was first passed in 1975 and was amended in 1997. To be eligible for special services under IDEA, a child must have a serious emotional disturbance, learning disabilities, mental retardation, traumatic brain injury, autism, vision or hearing impairment, or some other type of notable physical or health impairment. A multidisciplinary evaluation procedure is required to determine if a child is eligible for special education under IDEA; those who are eligible are subject to review at least once every three years. The evaluation team must also consider whether the child requires assistive technology devices or services.

IDEA guarantees special services for children not yet of school age who may need help with physical, cognitive, social, emotional, or adaptive development, as well as in communication areas. To be eligible for these services, children need to be evaluated by a special evaluation team.

Section 504

You might also hear the term "504" when school personnel talk about special services for children. Section 504 is a civil rights statute that is part of the Rehabilitation Act of 1973 and pertains to both public and private programs. It states that schools cannot discriminate against children with disabilities and must provide them with reasonable accommodations so they receive a fair and appropriate public education. Under the Section 504 provisions, anyone who has an impairment that limits learning or social development is considered disabled, and it is used especially for children and adolescents with ADHD. It typically includes low- or no-cost services such as untimed tests, seat assignments at the front of the class, or the ability to use a computer in the classroom. Children covered under Section 504 tend to have less severe disabilities than those who fall under IDEA.

The Americans with Disabilities Act

The Americans with Disabilities Act (ADA), passed in 1990, requires all educational institutions, other than those operated by religious organizations, to meet the needs of children with psychiatric and physical problems. It also prohibits the denial of educational services, programs, or activities to students with disabilities and prohibits discrimination against all such students.

Advocating for Your Child

While the legal aspects of providing your child with the services he or she needs are very important, equally valuable is developing a strong family-school bond so you and the teacher can communicate freely and comfortably in order to achieve the best results for your child. **Here are some suggestions that may help establish a good relationship:**

- **Meet with your child's teacher and discuss your concerns.** Teachers are often equally concerned and may welcome the opportunity to explore the best way to help your child.

- **Ask for written descriptions of what happens with your child in class.** This can be a formal letter or a notebook that travels from home to school. You can write about any concerns you have, and the teacher can note for you what is happening each day. These descriptions can also be an excellent way

for the teacher to remind you of what your child's homework focus should be.

- If the teacher advises, **give permission for your child to meet with the school psychologist.** Then set up a separate meeting to learn what you can from this professional.

- **Request a more formal evaluation of your child at any time.** All requests for evaluations and services should be made in writing and dated, and you should keep a copy of all such requests.

- If your child qualifies for an individualized education plan (IEP) or a 504 plan (explained more fully below), you should **play an active role in the preparation**. Keep all written observations by teachers, and copies of correspondence pertaining to your child. This record will be very helpful for future reviews and in the event of any disagreement about the services the school is obligated to provide. Both the IEP and the 504 plan are legal documents, so make certain that these are complete as possible .

- Remember that **the findings of the evaluation team are not final.** You have the right to appeal, and the school is required to provide you with the information about how to do so.

- **Parents and their children are guaranteed rights under federal and state laws.** If you become confused, check with the school or a child mental health advocacy group, such as Parents Helping Parents, about finding someone to help advocate for you.

- Whenever you can, **try to keep the situation with the school friendly.** If disputes arise, consider using mediation in addition to, or instead of, a full hearing.

A Proper Evaluation

If you've been in contact with school personnel about your child's issues, then the teacher or school psychologist may have already suggested having your child evaluated. A parent's suspicion that a child qualifies for special services is not enough to require the school to perform an evaluation. The decision to evaluate the child will be made by a school-based team, and they will make this decision only after being shown that a child is suffering academically because of a suspected disorder or disability.

If you, not the school, are making the request for an evaluation, the school will generally require that the request be made in writing. Date and keep all copies of such requests. If you're just starting out, devote a notebook to keeping track of all the paperwork related to your child's evaluation and special school services.

IDEA requires that the school district consider the findings of outside evaluators, and, in some cases, pay for independent evaluations. Parental consent is always required for IDEA evaluations. Although Section 504 requires nondiscriminatory testing, there are fewer regulations in place than with IDEA. I usually suggest that parents start with school evaluations. Many are remarkably thorough, and having the school perform the evaluation can save the family a great deal of money, since more and more insurance companies refuse to pay for educational testing. Most school districts will want to perform their own testing, anyway. Some school districts lack the funds or are so resistant to providing special educational services that they explicitly (or implicitly) encourage families to arrange for their own testing. If you decide to go this route, be aware that you will probably not receive any reimbursement for what can become several thousands of dollars.

If your child is evaluated by someone outside the school system, the school must still agree with the outsider's assessment, and a formal meeting will be called. Parents will be invited, but the meeting will happen whether you attend or not, so make an effort to attend. A counselor, one or more of your child's teachers, and the evaluation team will discuss whether, based on the evaluation, your child is eligible for special services.

If you disagree with the results of the

evaluation, refuse to sign anything that implies that you have accepted the findings of the evaluation process. Parents have the right to appeal their decision, and your school is legally required to provide you with information on how to appeal. If you doubt the original findings, this may be time to consider spending money on additional testing, as well as on a lawyer who specializes in these kinds of cases.

If the school deems your child eligible, then it will develop an individualized education program, or IEP, hopefully with your active cooperation. An IEP may provide anything from occupational or speech therapy to a personal classroom aide or special classroom. It can even stipulate that the school pay for having the child attend a private school with special services, if that is the best way to ensure that the child has an adequate environment in which to learn. A child's IEP must be reviewed annually, and the child must be reevaluated every three years.

About the IEP

While IDEA requires certain information be included in each child's IEP, the states and local school systems often include additional information documenting their compliance with certain aspects of federal or state law. As a result, there is some variation in the format of IEPs from state to state, and maybe even from school to school.

In general, most IEPs include the following:

- **Current performance.** The IEP must state how the child is currently doing in school. This information may include classroom tests and assignments, individual tests given to determine eligibility for services, or observations from teachers or school staff. The statement will include how the child's disability affects performance in school.

- **Annual goals.** These are goals the child can reasonably accomplish in a year. Often broken down into short-term objectives, the goals must be measurable so progress can be documented, and they may address academic, social, or behavioral issues.

- **Special education and related services.** The IEP must list services the child is to be provided. This may involve modifications to the program or support for school personnel that may require additional training in order to assist the child.

- **Participation with nondisabled children.** The IEP must explain the extent (if any) to which the child will not participate with nondisabled children in the regular classroom and other school activities.

- **Participation in state- and district-wide tests.** The IEP must stipulate what modifications will be made in order for the child to take any state or district achievement tests. If a test is not appropriate for a child, the IEP must state why the test is not appropriate and how the child will be alternately tested.

- **Dates and places.** The IEP must state when services will begin, how often and where they will be provided, and how long they will last.
- **Transition service needs.** Beginning when the child is age fourteen (or younger, if appropriate), the IEP must address, where applicable, the courses needed to reach post-school goals. A statement of transition services must also be included in each subsequent IEP.
- **Needed transition services.** Beginning when the child is age sixteen (or younger, if appropriate), the IEP must state what transition services are needed to help the child prepare for leaving school.
- **Age of majority.** Beginning at least one year before the child reaches the age of majority, the IEP must include a statement that the student has been informed of any rights that will transfer to him or her at the age of majority. This statement is only needed in states that transfer rights at the age of majority.
- **Measuring progress.** The IEP must state how the child's progress will be measured and how parents will be informed of that progress.

A Parent's Job

Though your child may have a legal right to special services, your job as a parent is to be certain that this right is recognized and appropriately carried out. As a result, keep the following in mind:

- Be proactive in learning about what your child is eligible for and being certain that level of services is being delivered.
- In general, it is best to assume the school and teacher are on your side and are there to be helpful. While you may find some individuals who are oppositional, for the most part, schools want what is best for the children and therefore, what is best for the classroom. Politeness, respect, and cooperation on your part is more likely to get you the best services for your child.
- If the school does not respond to your request or refuses services under IDEA or Section 504, you have the right to a due process hearing. Contact the U.S. Department of Education Office of Civil Rights Regional Office for assistance.

For more information on these programs, you can contact the National Dissemination Center for Children with Disabilities, your state's Department of Special Education, or the Office of Special Education within the U.S. Department of Education.

Early Intervention for the Young Child

Children with disabilities or behavioral disorders need services sooner, not later. The Individual with Disabilities Act provides that, when warranted, children under age five should be evaluated for possible problems. If an issue is found, then they are eligible for special services with the hope of giving them the support they need until they enter kindergarten when the school takes over that role.

If your child seems to be developing more slowly than other children, or if you have other reasons to believe that your child isn't developing normally, speak first with your pediatrician. He or she will be able to tell you if your concerns are warranted. If you continue to be concerned, keep asking the same question at each visit or ask for a second opinion. What might not concern a doctor when a baby is eighteen months old may make him or her suspicious when your child turns two and still hasn't reached a certain developmental milestone. If the pediatrician feels that further investigation is necessary, the pediatric office can provide you with information on having your child evaluated.

Developmental evaluations are available at no cost for children who are thought to be at risk. The Web site of the National Dissemination Center for Children with Disabilities, www.nichcy.org, also has helpful information, including state-by-state guides. You can also call the organization toll-free at 800-695-0285.

When you've found the appropriate state agency, explain that you have a young child you would like to have evaluated for early intervention services. This agency will refer you to the organization in your area who conducts these evaluations. Just as for school-aged children, IDEA requires that your child receive a timely, comprehensive, multidisciplinary evaluation and assessment to identify your child's strengths and weaknesses and to determine whether or not he or she is eligible for special services.

Following the evaluation, you will meet with a team of professionals to review the results. The team will discuss whether your child meets the criteria for IDEA and state policy for having a developmental delay, a diagnosed physical or mental condition, or is at risk for having any other sort of problem. If a child is found eligible for services, then an individualized family service plan (IFSP) will be created. This is a document that outlines plans and goals for supporting your child. Based on information available from the National Dissemination Center for Children with Disabilities' Web site, it may include:

- Your child's present physical, cognitive, communication, social, emotional, and adaptive developmental level and needs
- Family information (with your permission) including resources, priorities, and concerns
- The expected outcome for the child and family
- Specific services the child will receive, including everything from family training and counseling to occupational or physical therapy, speech therapy, audiology services, medical help for diagnostic purposes, health services as

needed, nutritional services, social work services, and assistive technology devices and services
- Time, location, and duration of services the child will receive (services for very young children are often provided in the home)
- Whether services provided are in a group or individual
- Name of the service coordinator
- Steps the family can take to support the child's transition out of early intervention services

Most services of this type are provided at no charge. However, there may be a sliding-scale charge depending on the rules of your state. In addition, some services may be covered by health insurance of Medicaid. Check with the contact person in your area to confirm any costs.

If You Move

If your family has to move to a new community or school district, your child still is guaranteed rights to the services previously provided. If you are moving to another state, you may find some variability in what the new school system can offer. However, if you work carefully with them, you will most likely be able to create a workable IEP method to provide the services your child requires. Still, be aware that moving late in the year or to a remote area with a low population of children can profoundly affect what services your child may receive. I've worked with families who spent months choosing their new location, with the final decision based largely on the types of services available for their children. As with anything, the more advance notice you have, the easier it will be to work out all the details. **Here are some points to remember:**

- In preparation for the move, check all of your child's records. If the IEP or IFSP is due soon, talk to your local school district (or for the IFSP, your local contact person) to see if an evaluation can be conducted early. Those who already know your child will be best prepared to gauge what may happen as a result of the move and write the IEP with that in mind. (This should be scheduled at least six weeks prior to the move in order to have the paperwork ready for the new district.) If your child is due for a triennial reevaluation, also try to take care of this in advance.
- Select one or more of the professionals or teachers that work with your child and ask them to write a letter containing any helpful information about your child for the new district, including strengths, weaknesses, and successful approaches to working with the child.
- If your child is due for a physical, try to get it done in advance and ask for your child's medical records, including a current list of immunizations and any information on past and current medication trials.
- If your child is taking regular prescription medicines, be sure to have at least a one-month supply and get copies of the prescriptions. If you need to see a doctor soon after the move, try to get a recommendation from your local doctor in advance and book the appointment before you move. There is nothing worse than trying to see a popular child psychiatrist only to learn that there is a long wait.
- Get in touch with the new school system, find a contact person, and schedule IEP meetings at the new school.
- Retain all the important records. While school information might be sent ahead if you have a specific contact at the new school, you don't want to risk losing any of this information. Don't pack it in your household moving boxes—keep it with the other important papers going directly with you.

When Your Child Nears Graduation

For a child with severe disabilities, most

states provide education and care until age twenty-one to twenty-three (Michigan maintains a program for young people up until age twenty-six). Several years before your child graduates, start learning all you can about laws regarding housing, medical care, and employment. A good place to start looking is the PACER Center in Minneapolis (www.taalliance.org), a national information center for families with disabled members.

Once your child is released from the public education program, parents should search for vocational and mental-health programs paid for by the state or covered by insurance. This often involves getting children on waiting lists.

If your child is relatively independent, you also must prepare yourself for this transition. Even parents of high-functioning children have trouble letting go, so don't feel upset if this is hard for you—it's hard for everybody. Once you've found the appropriate setting for your child, then it is time to let him or her try to make it alone.

The Bottom Line

As with many other topics discussed in this book, you will be challenged to become an expert on school structures and functions about which most parents remain ignorant. Where possible, you will want to ally yourself with good teachers and psychologists who know your child and the ways in which educational systems accommodate special needs. When that does not work, then you will need to assert yourself and be a staunch, but reasonable, advocate for your child's needs. Unfortunately, this is an ongoing task, and you will need to adapt to new demands and problems as your child advances through the school as well as through the many other aspects of development that affect your child's ability to function.

Ultimately, successful use of the school's resources is essential for the care of many children. If you encounter resistance from school officials, bear this in mind as it will be your reward when it works.

Chapter 15

Putting It All Together

Before writing this final chapter, I met with Josh's parents. Josh, nearly seven years old, has had a rough life. He was born prematurely, weighing slightly over two pounds. He spent the first several months of his life in a pediatric intensive care unit, and several more months after that at home with supplemental oxygen. Despite all that, he seemed physically fine, and his development progressed pretty unremarkably. Josh's parents noticed that his language was a bit delayed and odd at age two, but he seemed socially connected with them and bright, quickly recognizing letters and memorizing the books he loved to have read to him every evening. Then, at about age three-and-a-half, something went awry. His parents could recall no major dramatic events that set off the problem, but Josh began to grow frustrated, sometimes at the drop of a hat, and became aggressive toward other children or his parents. It didn't happen all that often, but often enough to cause his preschool teacher to suggest an evaluation.

An initial evaluation performed through the school showed mild language delay and some social withdrawal, but not enough to raise concern. He started speech and language therapy, which progressed well. The meltdowns continued periodically, usually set off by abrupt changes, such as making transitions from one task to another. His parents learned to let him know well in advance, when possible, about upcoming changes. They noted that although his vocabulary was superior for his age, they were often unsure if he understood them when they asked him a question. He also seemed to have little interest in his peers, although he liked playing with both older and younger children; the former liked to "parent" him, especially the girls, and the latter enjoyed having an older child who seemed to share their interests.

Because his birthday was in early December, Josh entered kindergarten just a few months before he turned six, yet the teacher noted that he was considerably less socially mature than his younger peers. He had the intellectual capacity to handle the material but was difficult behaviorally, often refusing to do tasks when asked and impulsively getting into trouble, especially with one aggressive boy in his class. He also had frequent tantrums when told to stop one task and begin another.

Another evaluation through the school revealed Josh had absolutely normal intellectual functioning with some skills and evidence of an auditory processing deficit—trouble not with hearing but with organizing and storing information that comes in through the ears as opposed to the eyes. Noting that Josh had few peer friends and was passionately interested in animals, the school psychologist also asked his parents to fill out a screening questionnaire for Asperger's disorder and, on the basis of a modestly high score on that questionnaire, suggested that Josh might have the disorder or some other form of PDD.

In the meantime, the family was working with a behavioral pediatrician. He had observed Josh at school and noted his impulsivity and physical restlessness, leading him to a suggestion of possible ADHD or anxiety. While admitting that he was uncertain about the diagnosis, the pediatrician felt that Josh's anxiety interfered with his function enough to suggest a SSRI trial. His parents agreed. Josh had no reaction the first few days on the medication

but after a week showed steady improvement, to the amazement of everyone. He became much less prone to outbursts, more able to tolerate transitions, and generally happier. This would have been perfect solution, except that the benefits gradually faded over the next few weeks, and the medicine was discontinued after about a month.

That was when Josh and his parents came to see me. His mother confided that when she had read about Asperger's disorder, she was sure that Josh had it; but, when she read about ADHD, she saw a lot of characteristics that seemed to fit her son as well. Josh's father was more skeptical that Josh had a problem at all, although his job kept him away from home for extended periods. Josh's mother, on the other hand, was at home full-time with Josh and his older sister.

Josh was much different in person than the testing suggested. He was bright, readily interactive, and seemingly fine. He did love animals of all kinds, but when he was speaking about them, he would check with me to see if I understood and he was willing to talk about other things when I showed signs of boredom. He showed no overt evidence of being hyperactive, impulsive, or even anxious most of the time. However, when I began asking him relatively simple questions, he initially failed to answer, then gave answers that suggested he wasn't sure of the question, and then began to demand that I stop talking to him because he was "tired" and "bored." An angry outburst soon followed.

Having reviewed the fairly extensive testing already done, obtaining a detailed history from Josh's parents, and meeting with the patient, I was ready to offer my opinion. I met with the parents, because I was pretty sure Josh would become upset and disruptive as we talked and did not believe that, in this instance, he needed to hear what I had to say. As happens much more frequently than I would like, I did not have the clear diagnosis and treatment recommendation for them I knew they were hoping "the expert" would provide. On the other hand, I thought I had a pretty good sense of why Josh was having trouble and what we could do to help him.

I began my summary by making sure that the parents and I saw Josh in the same way—not as a diagnosis but as a child. We discussed what I had heard and observed about them and Josh in terms of the sequence of events that led to problems, and I was pleased to confirm that they saw him in a quite similar way. I told Josh's father that things were more serious than he wanted to believe, and I told his mother that they were not as bad as she feared; I told both of them that it was important they work together. We discussed why Asperger's disorder and ADHD might fit

Josh's behavior and why I was sure neither diagnosis fit well enough to convince me. I also complemented them on the ways in which they had listened to Josh and created interaction styles with him that were clearly responsive to his needs for calm and clarity.

Then I offered them my explanation of Josh's problem. We started with his premature birth and intensive procedures afterwards. These may have had an effect on the way his brain formed and certainly affected his belief in the safety of the world, since he recurrently underwent a variety of procedures that were often distressing or painful. I noted that auditory processing problems are common, and perhaps more so in premature babies. I reminded his parents of my sense that Josh often did not understand what was said to him but tried to pretend he did, then suggested that most of his impulsive and oppositional behaviors and rages came when he was pushed to do something that he might not understand. If so, then his anxiety about transitions and unexpected events, even desirable ones, made sense: How could he know what might happen next?

Within that framework, we discussed Josh's one medication trial, the antidepressant that seemed to help initially but then stopped working or made him worse. In my experience, his initial response seemed real—it did not happen immediately, gradually grew over several days, and seemed consistent with a decrease in anxiety that allowed him to better tolerate change. He showed none of the later sleep or behavioral changes later that might suggest a manic response, so it is likely that either the deterioration was a result of a medication mismatch or improper dosage. Either possibility fit the facts, but the key was that he showed a positive response to medication, even if only briefly.

In short, I explained that Josh was not so much a traditional diagnosis as a word picture, called a formulation. Embedded in that description were some diagnoses, namely a language processing problem and anxiety disorder, but not a solitary explanation for his problems. His issues were integral components to a larger picture that included what we knew about biology, environment, and temperament.

Once we were agreed on this formulation, it was relatively easy to map out an intervention plan. We spoke primarily of nonmedication options, including ensuring that Josh was listening by having him stop, make eye contact, attend to instructions, and then repeat what he'd heard. His parents agreed to create a reward program based on his ability to repeat them accurately. We also discussed creating a calm intervention method, including brief timeouts, for dealing with Josh's rages. We talked about Josh acquiring better peer skills by starting out as a "big brother" to a younger child. I suggested that the role of medications, if there was one, would be to help Josh with the anxiety he experienced when faced with uncertainty. If all their efforts were thwarted by his anxiety, then we agreed to try a low dose of an antidepressant, with gradual increases if necessary to see if we could find a range that actually worked for Josh.

My Hope for You

It is my hope that those of you who have made it to this point in the book will have acquired the skills and knowledge needed to seek out someone who can help you construct a similar story about your child. If, as is my wife's wont with mystery novels, you started this book by skipping to the last few pages, then may what you read inspire you to start at the beginning, so you can learn how we got here.

In some ways, I cheated by using Josh and his family as an example, because no one knows how his story will turn out. Was I right in what I told his parents? Will the interventions we agreed upon actually produce the changes I predicted? We don't know yet. But you don't know about your situation, either. The concepts presented here are general ones. For your child, they may lead to significant changes, or perhaps none at all.

The purpose of this book is to assure you that what you are facing with your child is hard, but there are also many reasons for optimism. Ways exist to ease the burden for even the most severely ill children and adolescents, and knowledge about how to do that continues to expand.

Medications, if used well and wisely, are wonderful additions to the tools available for helping young patients. As with so many other aspects of the parenting role, your job is to learn enough to ensure that their use with your child truly is a step in the right direction toward a brighter future.

Administering Medications

Medicines never work if you don't take them. All too often, especially with younger children and patients with severe developmental delays, parents say, "So how do we do that?" This appendix, in part, is meant to acknowledge the many innovative ways parents have shared with me over the years of doing just that.

General Options

Psychoactive medications come in a variety of forms, and you should always ask your child's doctor about the available choices when you are considering a medication trial. For children who can swallow a pill, there are tablets, capsules, and caplets. Probably because so many more children are taking these medications, you may have the option of choosing a liquid form. For example, all of the SSRI antidepressants now come in liquid form. For some children, however, this turns out to be more problematic than the pill. A number of my patients are highly taste-sensitive and hate

the flavors provided. More recently, a few medications come as a quick-dissolving film—each dose is a flat sheet or porous-looking pill that dissolves almost instantly once placed on your tongue. These are being used especially in inpatient units with patients who pretend to take pills but then spit them out, but they can also be an alternative that some younger patients find fun and easy.

Rarely, you can get medicine into your child other than orally. For many years, clonidine (Catapres) was the only medicine commonly used that came as a patch worn on the back or shoulder, where the medicine is absorbed. A patch for methylphenidate (Ritalin) should soon be available.

Teaching Your Child to Swallow Pills

Most adults can swallow pills, leading to the conclusion that we learned how to do so at some point. For a child motivated to do so, learning to swallow a pill is not exceptionally difficult. In a study some years ago of seven- to nine-year-olds with ADHD, we had to train a number of children to swallow pills so they could be in the study. None of them had to drop out because they could not learn.

The general principle is to start small, reward success, and keep at it until you achieve the goal. It is best to treat the exercise like a game, if possible, and even better if you lead the way.

As with many lessons in life, the facts actually help. Humans have a wonderfully competent system for getting items from the mouth to the stomach, as evidenced every time we eat. This mechanism is so effective that you can stand on your head and still eat or drink, knowing that food and liquid will get to the stomach through a process called peristalsis. When an object hits the back of the throat, it stimulates a flap to cover the airway that leads to the lungs while initiating a series of rhythmic contractions of the esophagus, gently pushing the object all the way down to the stomach.

Why, then, can swallowing a pill be so hard? There are several reasons. Like walking, it can be harder to swallow if you're paying too much attention. Voluntary swallowing is sometimes out of sync with the automatic process. Also, if an object is too large or if we are convinced it is going to taste bad or we will not be able to swallow it, it can activate the gag reflex, a built-in safety device to keep unwanted objects out of the body. (My older son had a superb gag reflex when he was younger. Just looking at food he thought might taste bad was enough to cause it to engage, and we soon learned to stand to the side of him when introducing new foods.)

The trick is to make the process as automatic and free of unpleasant sensations as possible. You can do that by having the child stick out her tongue as far as possible, have her place the pill toward the back of the tongue (but not so far back that she touches her throat and gags), and then take a good swallow of a beverage of choice. To ensure success, start with something small, such as the edible silver balls used to decorate cakes. Once your child can swallow something that size, substitute a small candy. Once she succeeds with those, you probably are ready for the real thing.

Take your time. Demonstrate on yourself. Praise success and sympathize with failures. And remain confident.

If Swallowing Is Not an Option

If, despite your best efforts, swallowing is simply not going to happen (this often occurs with younger children and those with mental retardation or other developmental problems), there still is hope. As mentioned already, consider a liquid form, if one is available. Also, most of the sustained-release forms of stimulants are capsules that you can open and sprinkle the beads over a spoonful of applesauce or some other easily swallowed, small amount of food. Be sure to check with your doctor or pharmacist to make sure that the capsule can be opened by your child. For example, Concerta cannot be opened because its time-release properties depend on an intact capsule.

The following approach works only for medications that are relatively tasteless. Again, assuming you do not have a tablet with time-release properties and is not highly bitter, you can crush the prescribed dosage into a fine powder and mix it into any food your child likes. The key here is to keep the food-to-medicine ratio low, or your child may only get half the needed dose because he gets too full.

A riskier attempt is to put the crushed pill into a liquid. Often, you end up with a suspension, not a liquid, with an unknown amount of the medicine clumped in the bottom of the glass. Also, some medications may have little stability when exposed to liquids in that way, but it never hurts to ask. For example, fluoxetine (Prozac) was initially available in capsule form; it dissolved readily in most liquids

and was stable in the refrigerator for several weeks, making it easy to create a liquid preparation, especially for younger children who needed fairly small doses.

Some parents show a remarkable innovative streak for pills that are bitter and cannot be crushed. One of my favorites was a family whose child was taking an antidepressant available only in pill form. The mother discovered that one of her son's favorite sweets, a Rollo, was the perfect size to hold the daily pill inside the soft center. She would tuck it into the candy and give him his nightly treat, making sure he ate it all. Ironically, he regularly swallowed the much bigger candy but swore he could not down the pill. Other parents use chicken strips, cheese sticks, or meatballs. For children who like spicy or hot foods, the strong flavor may also help mask the taste.

Other Solutions

If you and your doctor are stuck, pharmacists can be of considerable help in these matters. Many pharmacies sell aides, including pill cutters and special plastic glasses, to facilitate pill swallowing. The glasses have a little cup built into the top edge of the glass. Put the pills in the cup, fill the glass with liquid, and then have the child take a big swallow with the small cup closest to the mouth. The idea is that the pills drop into the mouth and are carried to the back of the throat by the large amount of liquid.

Pharmacies also sometimes still have what are called formulating pharmacists. These individuals are trained to take medications and convert them into some other form, ranging from a liquid or suspension to a preparation designed to be absorbed through the skin. Be aware, however, that such preparations are not studied for absorption properties, so it may be hard to find the right dose or even know that your child actually is getting the medicine your doctor prescribed. Make sure the prescribing doctor knows about such special approaches so he or she can monitor the adequacy of treatment.

Resources

The following are resources you might find useful. It is by no means complete, and numbers and addresses may change at any time. Although I have not listed any organization whose motives or actions I find strongly objectionable, I do not intend inclusion to imply endorse-ment nor exclusion to imply criticism. What I do hope will be evident is that resources do exist. People just like you have faced problems similar to those you are struggling with and have tried to make the road a bit easier for the next person. May you do the same.

PROFESSIONAL ORGANIZATIONS

**American Academy of Child &
Adolescent Psychiatry**
3615 Wisconsin Avenue NW
Washington, DC 20016-3007
800-333-7636 or 202-966-7300
www.aacap.org

American Academy of Pediatrics
141 Northwest Point Boulevard
Elk Grove Village, IL 60007-1098
847-434-4000
www.aap.org

American Psychiatric Association
1000 Wilson Boulevard, Suite 1825
Alexandria, VA 22209-3901
888-357-7924 or 703-907-7300
www.psych.org

American Psychological Association
750 1st Street NE
Washington, DC 20002-4242
202-336-5510 or 800-374-2721
www.apa.org

**Association for Behavioral
and Cognitive Therapies**
305 7th Avenue, 16th floor
New York, NY 10001-6008
212-647-1890
www.aabt.org

Centers for Medicare & Medicaid Services
7500 Security Boulevard
Baltimore, MD 21244-1850
877-267-2323
www.cms.gov

National Institute of Mental Health (NIMH)
Office of Communications and
  Public Liaison
6001 Executive Boulevard
Room 8184, MSC 9663
Bethesda, MD 20892-9663
866-615-6464
Anxiety Disorders:
888-ANXIETY (888-269-4389)
www.nimh.nih.gov
nimhinfo@nih.gov

Psychology Today's Therapy Directory
(a searchable database for
  non-physician therapists)
http://therapists.psychologytoday.com/rms/
prof_search.php

Substance Abuse and Mental Health
  Services Administration
National Mental Health Information Center
P.O. Box 42557
Washington, DC 20015-0557
800-789-2647
www.mentalhealth.samhsa.gov

NATIONAL SELF-HELP AND SUPPORT ORGANIZATIONS

Anxiety Disorders Association of America
8730 Georgia Avenue, Suite 600
Silver Spring, MD 20910
240-485-1001
www.adaa.org

Autism Society of America
7910 Woodmont Avenue, Suite 300
Bethesda, MD 20814-3067
800-3AUTISM (800-328-8476) or
301-657-0881
www.autism-society.org

Children and Adults with Attention-
  Deficit/Hyperactivity Disorder (CHADD)
8181 Professional Place, Suite 150
Landover, MD 20785
301-306-7070
www.chadd.org

Depression and Bipolar Support Alliance
  (DBSA)
730 N. Franklin Street, Suite 501
Chicago, IL 60610-7224
800-826-3632 or 312-642-7243
www.dbsalliance.org

Freedom from Fear
308 Seaview Avenue
Staten Island, NY 10305-2246
718-351-1717 (ext. 24)
www.freedomfromfear.com

National Alliance on Mental Illness (NAMI)
Colonial Place Three
2107 Wilson Boulevard, Suite 300
Arlington, VA 22201-3042
703-524-7600
www.nami.org

National Mental Health Association
2001 N. Beauregard Street, 12th floor
Alexandria, VA 22311-1724
800-969-6642 or 703-684-7722
www.nmha.org

National Mental Health Consumers'
  Self-Help Clearinghouse
1211 Chestnut Street, Suite 1207
Philadelphia, PA 19107-4112
800-553-4539
www.mhselfhelp.org
info@mhselfhelp.org

Obsessive-Compulsive (OC)
  Foundation, Inc.
676 State Street
New Haven, CT 06511-6508
203-401-2070
www.ocfoundation.org
info@ocfoundation.org

SUICIDE PREVENTION OR DRUG OVERDOSE

Poison Control Hotline
800-222-1222
www.poison.org

National Hopeline Network
800-SUICIDE (800-784-2433)
www.hopeline.com

National Suicide Prevention Lifeline
800-273-TALK (800-273-8255)
www.suicidecepreventionlifeline.org

Acknowledgments

This volume was slow aborning and well might not have seen the light of day without Lynn Sonberg's belief in the project. I thank her for her perseverance in getting the process started, in facilitating the work at every step, and in keeping the pressure on until it was complete.

Kate Kelly deserves special and particular thanks for her pivotal contributions to the writing process. Kate was the perfect midwife, confidently guiding me through each step, offering both encouragement and perspective at each stage. I especially treasure the long talks we would have when a particular chapter was failing to gel, as I tried to clarify what I believed, and she reflected back what parents want to know.

My thanks go also to those at Stewart, Tabori & Chang for the care and attention they provided in turning the manuscript into a completed book. I am grateful especially for the efforts of Debora Yost, the acquiring editor, Christine Gardner, associate editor, and Andrea Glickson, the marketing director.

But, above all, I want to acknowledge the key role that my patients and their families have played. From them, I have learned the face, heart, and soul of mental disorders. In sharing a part of their lives with me, they have shown me the pain, confusion, and disruption that mental disorders can create; the love, laughter, and hope that can see them through the toughest times; and the hope and determination that keeps them moving toward the future.

Index

SSRIs, 96, 169, 172–73
and suicide,
20–21, 96, 168, 170, 173
tricyclic, 169, 171
antihistamines, 160, 216, 217
antipsychotics, 179–88
and anticonvulsants, 192, 196
atypical (second-generation),
182, 184–86
for children and
adolescents, 182
dosage of, 186–87
how they work, 181–83
reasons for using, 180, 185, 192
side effects of, 187–88
typical (first-generation),
182, 183–84
anxiety disorders, 100–123
and ADHD, 66
antianxiety drugs, 214–24
and bipolar disorder, 95
causes of, 103, 105
diagnosis of, 105, 118
generalized, 102–5, 217
living with, 101, 104, 220
obsessive-compulsive disorder,
114–16
panic disorder, 112–13
phobias, 107–10
post-traumatic stress disorder,
116–18
relaxation techniques for, 119
separation disorder, 105–7
and sleep problems, 222
social phobias, 110–12
symptoms of, 103
treatment of,
75, 105, 118–20, 168
what they are, 102–3

aplastic anemia, 184
applied behavior analysis
(ABA), 140
artificial sweeteners, 235
Asperger's disorder, 132–35
brain dysfunction in, 135
causes of, 135–36
diagnosis of, 50, 139–40
living with, 133–34, 165
as pervasive developmental
disorder, 134
symptoms of, 133
treatment of, 139–40
atomoxetine (Strattera), 210
attention span, increasing, 74
autism, 128–32
behavior modification for,
140–41
brain dysfunction in, 135
causes of, 135–36
diagnosis of, 128–30, 136, 139
increasing numbers of
cases, 132
language delays in,
129, 130–31
living with, 145–46
male-to-female ratio for, 135
miracle cures for, 147–48
odd behaviors in, 129–30, 132
outcome of, 130–31
as pervasive developmental
disorder, 134
and seizures, 143
severity of, 130
social isolation in, 129
splinter skills with, 131
treatment of,
139–41, 142, 144, 238

autism spectrum disorders,
132, 135
autistic savants, 131–32

B

barbiturates, 215
behavior:
abruptly starting, 30
analysis (ABA), 140
changes in, 84, 88
correcting, 40
criticizing, 40
dialectical therapy (DBT),
230–31
disorders, 58–81
disruptive, 143
food additives as cause of, 235
getting advice about, 30
inconsistent, 62
no recognizable cause for, 30
peculiar, 27, 129–30, 132, 133
perseverative, 142
persistent, 27
perturbing, 27–28
repetitive, 128, 142
ritualized, 146
targeted for therapy, 228–29
timing of, 27
videotapes of, 31, 53
behavioral approach, 119
behavior modification,
140–41, 228–29
benzodiazepines,
215, 216, 218, 222
benztropine (Cogentin), 180
beta-adrenergic antagonists,
215–16
beta-blockers, 215–16
Beth (trauma), 119